The Bath and Body Book

DIY Bath Bombs, Bath Salts, Body Butter and Body Scrubs

All Rights Reserved. No part of this publication may be reproduced in any form or by any means, including scanning, photocopying, or otherwise without prior written permission of the copyright holder. Copyright © 2014

Table of Contents

Bath Bombs
Introduction
BasicIngredients
What is Citric Acid and Where to Find It
Getting it Just Right
Molding the Bath Bombs

Bath Bomb Recipes
Basic Bath Bomb
Bath Bombs without Citric Acid Recipe
White Tea and Coconut Oil Bath Bomb Recipe
Water Softening Bath Bomb
Christmasy Bath Bombs
Dried Flower Bath Bombs
Easter Egg Bath Bombs
Bath Bomb Favors
Itty Bitty Bath Bombs
Green Tea Bath Bombs

Fortune Cookie Bath Bombs
Rustic Bath Bombs
Moisture Rich Bath Bombs
Fizzy Milk Bath Bombs
Shea Butter and Citrus Bath Bombs
Saturday Night Sizzle
Cinnamon Tea Bath Bombs
Hard as a Rock Bath Bombs
Manly Bath Bombs
Coconut and Vanilla Bath Bombs

Get Creative
Adding Extras
Molds
Tips and Considerations
Conclusion

Bath Salts
Introduction
Basic Ingredients
Borax? In Bath Salts?
Choosing the Right Ingredients

Bath Salts Recipes
Lavender Bath Salts
Eucalyptus and Vanilla Bath Salts
Rosemary Bath Salts
Simply Aromatherapy Bath Salts
Rainbow Bath Salts
Rose Milk Bath Salts
Two Ingredient Vanilla Bath Salts
Valentine's Day Bath Salt
Herbal Bath Salts
Moisturizing Bath Salts
Mint Mojito Bath Salts
Detoxifying Epsom Bath Salts
Orange Dreamsicle Bath Salts
Bath Salts for Back Pain

- [Lemon and Rosemary Bath Salts](#)
- [Grapefruit Bath Salts](#)
- [Simple Soothing Bath Salts](#)
- [Simple Re Relaxing Bath Salts](#)
- [A Simple Feel Good Bath Salt Mixture](#)
- [Sensual Bath Salts](#)
- [Uplifting Bath Salts](#)
- [Refreshing Bath Salts](#)
- [Energizing Bath Salts](#)
- [Extra Uplifting Bath Salts](#)
- [Bath Salts for Aches and Pains](#)
- [Tropical Bath Salts](#)
- [Bath Salts Tea Bag](#)
- [Fruitylicious Bath Salts](#)
- [Dead Skin Removing Bath Salts](#)
- [Autumn Orchard Bath Salts](#)
- [Couple's Bath Salts](#)
- [Easy To Make Bath Salt Blends in Bulk](#)
- [Himalayan Bath Salt Blends](#)
- [The Hangover Bath Salt Blend](#)
- [Bath Salt Blends for Men](#)

Bath Salt Blends for Kids
Bath Salts as Gifts
Conclusion

Body Butter
Introduction
Basic Ingredients and Tools
Storing the Body Butter
Shelf Life of Body Butter

Body Butter Recipes
Whipped Body Butter
White Chocolate Whipped Body Butter
Wild Rose Body Butter
Soothing Lavender and Mint Body Butter
Mint Chocolate Body Butter
Magnesium Body Butter
Mint Infused Coconut Body Butter
3-Ingredient Cocoa Body Butter
Coconut Oil and Honey Body Butter
Simple Mango Body Butter

- Coconut and Mango Body Butter
- 3-Ingredient Shea Body Butter
- Extreme Moisturizing Body Butter for Dry and Damaged Skin
- Hand Softener Body Butter
- Cocoa and Hemp Body Butter
- Aloe, Coconut and Lavender Body Butter
- Peppermint Tallow Whipped Body Butter
- Vanilla Bean Body Butter
- Anti-Bacterial Body Butter
- Key Lime Whipped Coconut Oil Body Butter
- Whipped Peppermint Body Butter
- Lavender Body Butter
- Rosemary Mint Body Butter
- Coconut & Rose Body Butter
- Cinnamon Body Butter for Cellulite
- Edible Chocolate Body Butter
- Coffee Body Butter Foot Cream
- Dreamy Lemon Cream Body Butter
- Super Glowy Body Butter

- Black Raspberry and Vanilla Body Butter
- The Simplest Body Butter
- The Wonderful Body Butter Recipe
- Sacred Frankincense Body Butter
- Ultra Moisturizing Body Butter
- Scrumptious Body Butter
- Shea and Coconut Body Butter
- Sugar Cookie Body Butter
- Honey Kissed Body Butter
- Sparkling Citrus Mango Body Butter
- Lavender Spice Body Butter
- Lavender Flower Body Butter
- Body Butter To Die For
- Manly Body Butter
- White Chocolate and Peppermint Body Butter
- Sweet Citrus and Vanilla Body Butter
- Lavender and Vanilla Body Butter
- 2-Ingredient Coconut and Vanilla Body Butter
- Bellby Butter for Pregnancy

Body Butter for Eczema
Coconut and Plum Body Butter
Body Butter Bars
Tips and Considerations
Conclusion

Body Scrubs
Introduction
Start Your Journey Here
Arm Yourself: The Tools and Ingredients Needed to make your Body Scrub a Hit
Sweet or Salty: The Difference Between Sugar -Body Scrubs and Salt Body Scrubs

The Recipes
For the Newbie: Simple and Easy Body Scrub Recipes for Beginners
Mind, Body and Soul: Homemade Body Scrubs for Health and Well Being
Sugar, Spice and Everything Nice: Body

[Scrub Recipes for Women](#)
[Snips and Snails and Puppy Dog Tails: Body Scrub Recipes for Men](#)
[For the Little Ones: Body Scrubs Safe for Children](#)
[Changing with the Season: Holiday Themed and Seasonal Body Scrub Recipes](#)
[Kissable and Lickable: Homemade Scrub Recipes for Lips](#)
[Put your Best Face Forward: Homemade Facial Scrub Recipes](#)
[Don't Forget the Feet: Recipes for Homemade Foot Scrubs](#)
[How to Use Body Scrubs](#)

[Gift Giving](#)
[Shelf Life: Prolonging the Shelf Life of your Homemade Body Scrubs](#)
[Storage: Choosing the Right Container for Body Scrubs](#)

The Devil is in the Detail: Prepare the Body Scrubs for Presentation Conclusion

Bath Bombs

Introduction

My family is rather large and filled with aunts and uncles, nieces and nephews, cousins and those twice removed. And while I love having a large family, it can be nerve racking and a bit expensive when the holiday season rolls around. At one point, I began baking cookies as gifts. Not only did it save me money, but also I was able to reduce a bit of stress since I didn't have to go from store to store trying to find gifts for everyone. Unfortunately, the cookie debacle of 2006 (as it has since become known) ended up with my uncle spending time in the emergency room because of some rather delicious chocolate chip cookies that I made with a bit of cinnamon to spice them up. Now how was I supposed to know he was deathly allergic to cinnamon?

So it was back to the drawing board to think of something else I could do. I didn't want to continue to bake knowing that I couldn't possibly remember who was allergic to what and I didn't want to take the chance of someone else having a bad experience with my cooking. So I began scoured the internet and craft books trying to find something else I could make as gifts. I thought about crocheting, but my Grandmother was the crocheter of the family and there was no way I could rival her skills.

After what seemed like weeks, I finally stumbled upon bath bombs. Bath bombs are these nifty little things that you toss in your bath. They create a foamy, bubbly action that can help relax tired muscles and leave your skin feeling soft and refreshed. Besides being easy to make and very budget-friendly, one of the great thing about bath bombs is that, despite the popularity of homemade gifts, there probably won't be another member of you family making them to give out as presents. Bath bombs are also very versatile, which means you can make them to fit anyone's personal needs, taste and style. For example, my older female cousin loves seashells and her bathroom has a pink color scheme, while her daughter loves cats and the color peach. Taking that into consideration, I was able to make them both seashell and cat-shaped bath bombs in the coordinating colors.

I began making bath bombs as Christmas presents in 2007, and they were -- and still are -- a hit! My family members actually look forward to receiving them, and have even called me up in the middle of the year asking if I could give them a few more bath bombs to hold them off until the holiday season rolls around.

Basic Ingredients

While every bath bomb recipe varies from one another, there are a few common and basic ingredients that are necessary to successfully create bath bombs; baking soda and citric acid. However, even the basic ingredients of bath bombs may vary depending on the recipe you use. For instance, some people have a hard time finding citric acid so there are a few recipes for bath bombs that don't require the use of citric acid. Keep in mind, however, that it is the citric acid -- along with the baking soda -- that creates those wonderful bubbles when the bath bomb is added to water. The alternative recipes -- which will be discussed later -- will work, just usually not as well as bath bombs that contain citric acid.

What is Citric Acid and Where to Find It

Most of the ingredients for bath bombs are relatively easy to obtain, except for citric acid. Citric acid is a natural product and is what gives lemons their sour taste. In fact, citric acid is used in various products and process. It is often used in cannoning as a preservative and it's used for cleaning and water softening. Consider looking for citric acid near the canning section of your local grocery store. You can also check with the health food store in your area since they may carry it in bulk. Citric acid is sometimes called 'sour salt', so you may have to use that terminology when searching for the item. Another option is to simply purchase citric acid from one of the many online merchants who carry it.

Getting it Just Right

One of the most important aspects of successfully creating bath bombs is achieving the right consistency. This is actually the trickiest part of the entire process. Once you have it down, however, creating bath bombs will be a breeze. What's so problematic is that every little thing can have an effect on the mixture. Every type of fragrance oil reacts differently to the bath bomb mixture, and even the weather can negatively impact the bath bomb making process. Yep, you read that correctly: The humidity level can actually affect the bath bombs and make it difficult to achieve the right consistency. The perfect consistency for bath bombs is like damp sand that you can pack together with your hands.

If the mixture is too wet, it will:

- Feel like doughy like Play-Doh, sticks to your fingers
- Feel overly wet

If the mixture is too dry, it will:

- Be crumbly, hard or pebbly
- Feel like dry sand that slips through your fingers
- Clump together only for a few seconds before crumbling apart

If the bath bomb is too wet, you can try adding a bit more of the prepared dry mixture to it. However, you should ensure it keeps the proper ratio of 2 parts sodium and 1 part citric acid. Having too much or too little of the sodium or acid will affect on how fizz the bath bombs produce. If the mixture is too dry, simply add a bit more of the liquid ingredients to the dry.

Molding the Bath Bombs

While it may sound simple enough, adding the mixture to the mold can be a bit tricky. This is due to the fact that the mixture has to be tightly packed into the mold. To properly mold the bath bombs you should spoon a bit of the mixture into the mold and then pack it in tightly with your fingers or the back of the spoon. Add a bit more mixture and pack again. Continue in this manner until you have filled the entire mold with the mixture.

Bath Bomb Recipes

Basic Bath Bomb

This first recipe

Ingredients:

- 2 cups of baking soda
- 1 cup citric acid
- 1 cup Epsom salt
- 1 teaspoon water
- 3 tablespoons light vegetable oil

Directions:

Step 1: Mix the dry ingredients together in a bowl.

Step 2: Mix the liquid ingredients in

Step 3: Slowly add the dry and liquid ingredients together, mixing together with a whisk. The mixture should have the consistency of damp sand, clumping together when squeezed into a ball.

Bath Bombs without Citric Acid Recipe

Ingredients:

- 2 cups baking soda
- 1/2 cup cream of tartar
- Water
- Essential oil (optional)
- Food color (optional)

Directions:

Step 1: Combine the baking soda and cream of tartar together. Add the essential oil and color if desired, and mix thoroughly.

Step 2: Add 1 teaspoon of water at a time, mixing after each one is added, until you can squeeze the mixture in your hand and it clumps together. If the clump begins to fall apart, you need to add a bit more water.

Step 3: Press the bath bomb mixture into the molds, making sure it is packed very tightly and let set for a few minutes. Gently tap the bath bombs out of the mold and let them dry overnight.

White Tea and Coconut Oil Bath Bomb Recipe

Ingredients:

- 1/2 cup cornstarch
- 1 cup baking soda
- 1/2 cup citric acid
- 2 tablespoons Epsom salts
- 2 tablespoons coconut oil
- 5 teaspoons of strong white tea (water can be used as a substitute)
- Few drops of the essential oil of your choosing, optional
- All-natural food coloring, optional
- Mold
- Airtight container

Directions:

Step 1: Mix cornstarch, baking soda, citric acid and Epsom salts together in a large bowl. Use a whisk to work the coconut oil in to the dry ingredients. Continue until the mixture becomes sandy with some chunks of oil.

Step 2: Add the white tea to the dry ingredients 1 teaspoon at a time, making sure to immediately stir with a large wooden spoon after each teaspoon is added. Keep in mind that the mixture will foam up a bit after each teaspoon of liquid added. This is normal and nothing to be concerned about.

Step 3: Continue stirring until the mixture has the same texture and appearance as sand that is slightly damp. You are ready to proceed to the next step when the mixture is primarily dry but can stick together when you squeeze some between your hands.

Step 4: When you are ready to continue, simply press the bath bomb mixture into the mold. The mixture was be tightly and firmly packed into the mold. Set the mold in a safe location to dry for at least 4 hours but preferably overnight. After the allotted time has passed, carefully remove the bath bombs from the mold and place in an airtight container until you are ready to use.

Water Softening Bath Bomb

Ingredients:

- 1 cup baking soda
- 1/2 cup citric acid
- 1/2 cup cornstarch
- 2 1/2 tablespoons oil
- 3/4 tablespoon water
- 2 teaspoons essential oil
- 1/2 teaspoon borax
- Cookie sheet

Directions:

Step 1: Mix the baking soda, citric acid and cornstarch together in a clean bowl.

Step 2: Mix oil, water, essential oil and borax together in a separate bowl.

Step 3: Slowly add the wet ingredients to the dry ingredients, using one hand to squish the ingredients together.

Step 4: Tightly pack the bath bombs into the molds. Let sit for a minute or two and then flip the molds over and carefully tap the bath bombs onto a cooking sheet. Let them dry overnight.

Christmasy Bath Bombs

Ingredients:

- 8 ounces baking soda
- 4 ounces citric acid
- 4 ounces cornstarch
- 4 ounces Epsom salts
- 3/4 teaspoon water
- 2 teaspoons peppermint essential oil
- 2.5 teaspoons light oil (such as almond oil)
- Red food coloring
- Fillable clear plastic ball ornament
- Cookie sheet
- Wax paper

Directions:

Step 1: Mix the dry ingredients together in a bowl.

Step 2: Mix the liquid ingredients in a small bowl.

Step 3: Pour the liquid mixture into the dry mixture and stir with a whisk. The mixture

Step 4: Tightly pack the mixture into half of the ornament. Do the same with the second half.

Step 5: Add a little more of the mixture on top of the second half of the ornament. Press the two halves together. If the mixture isn't packing well, simply place it back into the bowl and slowly add a little bit of water at a time. Remember, too much water will ruin the bath bomb.

Step 6: After a few minutes, carefully remove the bath bomb from the mold. Set the bath bombs on a clean cookie sheet lined with wax paper and allow to dry for at least 24 hours.

Dried Flower Bath Bombs

Ingredients:

- 2 cups baking soda
- 1 cup citric acid
- 1 cup cornstarch
- 1/2 teaspoon essential oil of your choosing
- 1 to 3 teaspoons olive oil
- Dried flower
- 5 drops food coloring
- Water-filled spray bottle
- Round mold

Directions:

Step 1: Mix the dry ingredients in a medium-size bowl.

Step 2: Mix the essential oil and olive oil together in a small bowl. Add the food coloring and mix thoroughly.

Step 3: Add the oils slowly to the dry ingredients, stirring until well mixed.

Step 4: Mist the mixture with the water until it begins to feel like wet sand and can be packed together.

Step 5: Pack the bath bomb mixture into the round mold, making sure it is packed as tightly as possible.

Step 6: Wait a few minutes and then carefully turn the mold over and tap the bath bomb out.

Step 7: Let the bath bombs stand for 1 to 2 days until thoroughly dry.

Easter Egg Bath Bombs

Ingredients:

- 6 tablespoons almond oil
- 4 teaspoons lavender essential oil
- 3 tablespoons water
- 8 ounces citric acid powder
- 8 ounces cornstarch
- 8 ounces cornstarch
- Food coloring
- Glitter
- Plastic Easter eggs
- Fluffy towel
- Baking sheet
- Wax paper

Directions:

Step 1: Combine the dry ingredients together in a large mixing bowl.

Step 2: Whisk the almond oil, lavender essential oil and water together in a smaller bowl.

Step 3: Add food coloring to the wet ingredients one drop at a time until you reach the desired coloring.

Step 4: Slowly add the wet ingredients to the dry ingredients. Mix together with your hands. The mixture should have a moist, sandy texture that clumps together in your hand.

Step 5: Fill the Easter eggs with the mixture packing it tightly. Allow the mixture-filled mold to sit for several minutes.

Step 6: Place a clean, fluffy towel over a baking sheet. Place a sheet of wax paper on top of the fluffy towel. The towel helps prevent the Easter egg bath bombs from becoming flat on the bottom.

Step 7: Remove the bath bombs carefully from the Easter egg mold. Place them safely on the baking sheet and let dry for about 2 days.

Bath Bomb Favors

DIY bath bombs make a great bridal or wedding favor that is both economical and easy to complete. You can even get your bridesmaids, family members and friends to help you make them.

Ingredients:

- 1 cup baking soda
- 1/2 cup citric acid
- Spray bottle filled with witch hazel
- Essential oil or fragrance oil of your choosing
- Water free colorant
- Mini-muffin pan
- Wax paper

Directions:

Step 1: Mix the baking soda and citric acid together in a bowl with a whisk, making sure to break up any clumps.

Step 2: Add the desired essential oil or fragrance oil to the dry mixture one or two drops at a time. The amount needed varies depending on the type of oil you are using and how strong of a scent you want. Continue adding one to two drops at a time, stirring and smelling the mixture after every drop until you reach the desired scent.

Step 3: Add the water-free colorant one drop at a time to the mixture, stirring after each drop. If any clumps form, use your fingers to break them up.

Step 4: Spritze the mixture with witch hazel until the dry ingredients can be clumped together in your hand.

Step 5: Pack the mixture into the muffin tin. Make sure to press the mixture tightly into the muffin tin.

Step 6: Let the muffin tin sit for 10 minutes. During this time, lay a sheet of wax paper on top of a cookie sheet.

Step 7: Turn the muffin tin over and carefully tap the bottom of the tin to encourage the bath bombs to carefully fall out and onto the wax paper.

Step 8: Allow the bath bombs to dry overnight. When dry, carefully package them in small wedding favor boxes topped with a ribbon, the bride and groom's name and wedding date.

Itty Bitty Bath Bombs

Ingredients:

- 1 cup baking soda
- 1/2 cup citric acid
- 1/2 cup cornstarch
- 1 tablespoon baby oil
- 1/2 teaspoon witch hazel
- 1 teaspoon essential oil
- Food coloring
- Silicone ice cube mold

Directions:

Step 1: Whisk the dry ingredients together in a bowl.

Step 2: Whisk the baby oil, witch hazel and essential oil together.

Step 3: Add one drop of food coloring at a time to the liquid ingredients. Stir after each drop. Continue until you have achieved the desired color.

Step 4: Add the liquid ingredients to the dry ingredients a little at a time, quickly stirring after each bit is added.

Step 5: Continue adding the liquid ingredients until the dry ingredients have the same consistency as damp sand and you can clump the mixture together in your hand.

Step 6: Pack the mixture tightly into the silicone ice tray mold. Let sit for at least 4 hours but preferably overnight.

Step 7: Carefully remove the bath bombs from the ice cube tray and store in an airtight container until ready to use.

Green Tea Bath Bombs

Ingredients:

- 2 tablespoons baking soda
- 1 tablespoon citric acid
- 1 tablespoon cornstarch
- 1 tablespoon Epsom salts
- 1/4 teaspoon canola oil
- 3/4 teaspoon strong green tea
- 1 or 2 drops of green food coloring

Directions:

Step 1: Brew a strong cup of green tea and let cool to room temperature.

Step 2: While the tea is cooling, whisk together the baking soda, citric acid, cornstarch and Epsom salts in a medium-sized bowl.

Step 3: Mix 3/4 teaspoon of the cooled green tea with 1/4 teaspoon of canola oil and 1 to 2 drops of green food coloring.

Step 4: Slowly pour the wet ingredients into the dry ingredients, whisking while you pour.

Step 5: Continue whisking until the mixture begins to resemble damp sand. When you can clump the mixture in your hand, you are ready for the next step.

Step 6: Spoon the bath bomb mixture into the mold. Press the mixture tightly into the mold.

Step 7: Let the bath bombs sit for about 4 hours before popping them out and allowing them to dry completely for 1 to 2 days.

Fortune Cookie Bath Bombs

Ingredients:

- 8 ounces baking soda
- 4 ounces citric acid
- 4 ounces cornstarch
- 4 ounces salts, such as Dead Sea salts, mineral salts or Epsom salts
- 3/4 tablespoon water
- 2 tablespoons essential or fragrance oil
- 2 1/2 tablespoons light oil
- 1 to 2 drops of food coloring
- Fortune cookie mold

Directions:

Step 1: Mix together the dry ingredients ensuring that all lumps and clumps are removed.

Step 2: Blend the liquid ingredients together in a small jar. If the jar has a lid, you can simply place the lid on top of the jar and shake for several seconds to thoroughly combine the wet ingredients.

Step 3: Slowly add the wet ingredients to the dry ingredients while whisking. If the mixture begins to foam, you are adding the liquid too quickly. Slow down and remember to keep whisking.

Step 4: Once you have added and mixed the wet and dry ingredients together, it should squish into a clump in your hand.

Step 5: Press the bath bomb mixture into the fortune cookie mold. Let sit for several minutes before popping the bath bombs out of the mold and onto a wax paper-covered cookie sheet.

Step 6: Allow the bath bombs to dry for 24 to 48 hours in a cool, dry location at of direct sunlight and away from direct heat.

Rustic Bath Bombs

Ingredients:

- 10 ounces baking soda
- 6 ounces granulated citric acid
- 6 ounces cornstarch
- 6 ounces Epsom salts finely grounded
- 4 teaspoons water, divided
- 4 to 8 teaspoons essential oil, divided
- 4 teaspoons extra virgin coconut oil, divided
- Food coloring (optional)
- Dried herbs and dried flowers
- Plastic Easter egg mold
- Empty egg carton

Directions:

Step 1: Combine the baking soda, citric acid, cornstarch and Epsom salts together in a large bowl. Whisk the ingredients together.

Step 2: Decide how many different bath bomb scents you want to use for this batch. This recipe typically makes 12 eggs, so divide the dry ingredients accordingly into separate bowls. For example, if you want 4 different scents, divide the dry ingredients by 7 ounces into 4 separate bowls. If, however, you are only using 1 scent, just use one large bowl.

Step 3: For my rustic bath bombs, I used 4 different scents, so I set out 4 bowls and filled each one with 1 teaspoon of water, 1 to 2 drops of food coloring, 1 to 2 teaspoons of essential oil and 1 teaspoon of coconut oil. Mix the liquid ingredients together.

Step 4: Slowly add the wet ingredients to the dry, mixing with a whisk. The mixture will begin to bubble a little and clump together. When this happens, set the whisk aside and begin using your fingers to work the mixture together.

Step 5: If the plastic Easter eggs have a small piece of plastic that attaches the two halves together, snip it off with a pair of scissors.

Step 6: Place dried herbs and/or dried flowers in the top half of the plastic Easter egg.

Step 7: Fill both halves of the Easter eggs with the mixture, packing it in as tightly as possible.

Step 8: Add a little bit of mixture to the top of one half of the egg. Press the two halves together.

Step 9: Set the plastic eggs up right inside an egg carton. Let sit for 10 minutes.

Step 10: Carefully invert the plastic egg and remove the bottom half by gently squeezing and twisting until it comes off.

Step 11: Place the inverted egg with the top half still attached back into the carton. Let the eggs dry for about 2 to 4 hours.

Step 12: Carefully place the bottom half back on the egg, and remove the top half in the same manner as you removed the bottom half.

Step 13: Gently place the egg-shaped bath bomb back into the egg carton and let dry for another 4 hours.

Step 14: Lay a plush, soft towel out on a flat surface where the bath bombs will not be disturbed. Carefully lay the bath bombs on the towel and let dry overnight. In humid areas, it may take up to 2 days for the bath bombs to dry completely.

Tips: If you want to forgo the Easter egg shape, simply line a muffin pan with paper cups and press the mixture tightly into the cavities of the pan. Let sit for 2 hours before removing the cups and letting the bath bombs dry on a fluffy towel for 24 hours.

Moisture Rich Bath Bombs

Ingredients:

- 1 cup baking soda
- 1/2 cup cornstarch
- 1/4 cup Epsom salt
- 1/2 cup citric acid
- 2 3/4 tablespoons almond oil
- 3/4 tablespoon water
- 1/4 teaspoon borax
- 1 1/2 teaspoon essential oil or fragrance oil
- Colorant
- Mold

Directions:

Step 1: Whisk the dry ingredients together.

Step 2: Combine the wet ingredients in a separate bowl.

Step 3: Add the wet ingredients to the dry ingredients while whisking together.

Step 4: Press the mixture tightly into the mold and let sit for 5 to 10 minutes.

Step 5: Remove the bath bombs from the mold and set on a fluffy towel.

Step 6: Let the bath bombs dry overnight.

Fizzy Milk Bath Bombs

Ingredients:

- 1 cup baking soda
- 1/2 cup citric acid
- 1/2 cornstarch
- 1/3 Epsom salts, finely grounded
- 1/4 cup powdered milk
- 2 tablespoons olive oil
- 2 teaspoons cocoa butter, melted
- 1 teaspoon essential or fragrance oil
- Distilled water
- Witch hazel
- Spray bottle
- Mold

Directions:

Step 1: Mix a 50/50 ratio of distilled water and witch hazel in the spray bottle. Set aside for the moment.

Step 2: Mix the dry ingredients together in large bowl. Make sure to mix out any lumps.

Step 3: Slowly drizzle the olive oil, melted butter and essential or fragrance oil over top the dry mixture.

Step 4: Use your hands to work the wet ingredients into the dry ingredients.

Step 5: Mist the mixture lightly with the distilled water and witch hazel solution. Mix once again with your hands.

Step 6: Continue misting the mixture lightly and mixing with your hands until you achieve the consistency of damp sand that easily clumps together.

Step 7: Pack the bath bomb mixture into the mold tightly. Let sit for 5 to 10 minutes.

Step 8: Carefully remove the bath bombs from the mold and place on a cookie sheet lined with wax paper.

Step 9: Allow the bath bombs to dry for 24 to 48 hours before storing them in an airtight glass jar.

Shea Butter and Citrus Bath Bombs

Ingredients:

- 1 cup baking soda
- 1/2 cup citric acid
- 1 tablespoon Shea butter, melted
- 3 milliliters grapefruit essential oil
- 1/2 milliliter of waterless colorant, such as LaBomb colorant
- 3 spritzes of water
- Stainless steel mold

Directions:

Step 1: In a large, clean mixing bowl, combine the dry ingredients together. Use a wire whisk to thoroughly combine the ingredients and break up any lumps that appear.

Step 2: Drizzle the melted Shea butter, grapefruit essential oil and waterless colorant over the dry ingredients. Blend together with your hands.

Step 3: Spritze the ingredients about 3 times with water, mixing with your hands after each spritze. Continue until you can clump the mixture together in your hand.

Step 4: Scoop the mixture into the stainless steel mold, pressing the mixture tightly into the mold.

Step 5: Let sit for a few minutes before removing the bath bombs from the stainless steel mold and placing on a cookie sheet lined with wax paper.

Step 6: Place the cookie sheet in a safe, cool and dry location away from direct heat and out of direct sunlight. Let the bath bombs dry for 1 to 2 days.

Saturday Night Sizzle

Ingredients:

- 10 tablespoons baking soda
- 2 1/2 tablespoons cornstarch
- 2 tablespoons tapioca starch
- 5 tablespoons citric acid
- 1 1/2 tablespoons canola or sweet almond oil
- 1/2 teaspoon sodium lauryl sulfoacetate
- 2 to 3 drops of soap colorant
- 1 tablespoon essential or fragrance oil
- Witch hazel

Directions:

Step 1: Sieve the dry ingredients together and into a large mixing bowel.

Step 2: Mix the oil, sodium lauryl sulfoacetate, colorant and essential or fragrance oil together.

Step 3: Pour the liquid over the dry ingredients and mix together with your hands.

Step 4: Spray the witch hazel lightly over the mixture and work it into the mixture. Continue lightly spraying the mixture with the witch hazel and mixing with your hands until it has the texture of damp sand.

Step 5: Press the mixture into the mold and let sit for a few minutes.

Step 6: Remove the bath bomb from the mixture and place on a cookie sheet covered with a fluffy towel. Allow the bath bombs to dry for 24 hours.

Lotsa Variations Bath Bombs

Ingredients:

- 1/2 cup baking soda
- 2 tablespoons citric acid
- 2 tablespoons sodium lauryl sulfoacetate
- 1 tablespoons tapioca starch
- 2 tablespoons Shea butter, melted
- 5 drops each of peppermint, sage and lavender essential oil
- Witch hazel

Directions:

Step 1: Pour witch hazel into a clean spray bottle. Set off to the side.

Step 2: Mix the dry ingredients in a clean mixing bowl.

Step 3: Combine melted Shea butter and the essential oil together in a small bowl.

Step 4: Drizzle the melted Shea butter and oil mixture over top the dry ingredients. Use your hands to work the ingredients into one another.

Step 5: Spray the mixture with witch hazel until you can clump it together in your hands.

Step 6: Press the damp sand-like mixture into the desired molds, letting it rest for a few minutes.

Step 7: Turn the mold upside and carefully tap the bath bombs out of the mold.

Step 8: Set the bath bombs on a cookie sheet lined with wax paper and let harden for 24 to 48 hours.

Cinnamon Tea Bath Bombs

Ingredients:

- 2 tablespoons baking soda
- 1 tablespoon citric acid
- 1 tablespoon cornstarch
- 1 tablespoon Epsom salts
- 1/4 teaspoon canola oil
- 3/4 teaspoon strong cinnamon tea
- 1 or 2 drops of red food coloring

Directions:

Step 1: Brew a strong cup of cinnamon tea and let cool to room temperature.

Step 2: While the tea is cooling, whisk together the baking soda, citric acid, cornstarch and Epsom salts in a medium-sized bowl.

Step 3: Mix 3/4 teaspoon of the cooled cinnamon tea with 1/4 teaspoon of canola oil and 1 to 2 drops of red food coloring.

Step 4: Slowly pour the wet ingredients into the dry ingredients, whisking while you pour.

Step 5: Continue whisking until the mixture begins to resemble damp sand. When you can clump the mixture in your hand, you are ready for the next step.

Step 6: Spoon the bath bomb mixture into the mold. Press the mixture tightly into the mold.

Step 7: Let the bath bombs sit for about 4 hours before popping them out and allowing them to dry completely for 1 to 2 days.

Hard as a Rock Bath Bombs

Ingredients:

- 1 cup baking soda
- 1/2 cup citric acid
- 1/4 cup Kaolin clay, also known as cosmetic clay
- 1/4 cup sugar
- 1 large Vitamin E oil capsule, or 2 small capsules
- 2 1/2 tablespoons olive oil
- 1 tablespoon skin safe fragrance oil or 20 drops essential oil
- 3 teaspoons water
- Colorant

Directions

Step 1: Mix the baking soda, citric acid and clay together in a large mixing bowl.

Step 2: Add one to two drops of the colorant to the dry mixture and knead with your hands.

Step 3: Add the water, olive oil and fragrance or essential oil into a spray bottle. Pierce the vitamin E capsule and dump the contents into the spray bottle.

Step 4: Secure the lid on the spray bottle and shake vigorously for several seconds.

Step 5: Spray the dry ingredients with the liquid 1 to 2 times, kneading the mixture with your hand after every spray. Continue spraying and kneading until the mixture has a consistency of damp sand that you can clump together.

Step 6: Tightly pack the mixture into the desired mold. Wait a minute or two before tapping them out of the mold and onto a wax paper-lined cookie sheet.

Step 7: Set the cookie sheet in a dry location and let air dry for 24 hours.

Manly Bath Bombs

Ingredients:

- 2 tablespoons baking soda
- 1 tablespoon citric acid
- 1 tablespoon cornstarch
- 1 tablespoon Epsom salts
- 1/4 teaspoon coconut oil
- 3/4 teaspoon strong coffee
- Coffee grounds and walnuts, finely grounded
- Mini muffin tin

Directions:

Step 1: Brew a strong cup of coffee and let cool to room temperature.

Step 2: While the coffee is cooling, whisk together the baking soda, citric acid, cornstarch and Epsom salts in a medium-sized bowl. Add the finely grounded coffee grounds and walnuts to the mixture.

Step 3: Mix 3/4 teaspoon of the cooled coffee with 1/4 teaspoon of coconut oil.

Step 4: Slowly pour the wet ingredients into the dry ingredients, whisking while you pour.

Step 5: Continue whisking until the mixture begins to resemble damp sand. When you can clump the mixture in your hand, you are ready for the next step.

Step 6: Spoon the bath bomb mixture into the mini muffin tin. Press the mixture tightly into the muffin tin cavity.

Step 7: Let the manly bath bombs sit for about 4 hours before popping them out of the mini muffin tin and allowing them to dry completely for 1 to 2 days.

Coconut and Vanilla Bath Bombs

Ingredients:

- 2 tablespoons baking soda
- 1 tablespoon citric acid
- 1 tablespoon cornstarch
- 1 tablespoon Epsom salts
- 1/4 teaspoon canola oil
- 1/4 teaspoon vanilla extract
- 1/4 teaspoon coconut extract
- 1 or 2 drops of blue skin-safe colorant

Directions:

Step 1: Whisk together the baking soda, citric acid, cornstarch and Epsom salts in a medium-sized bowl.

Step 3: Mix the vanilla extract, coconut extra, canola oil and 1 to 2 drops of blue colorant together in a small bowl.

Step 4: Drizzle the wet ingredients slowly over the dry ingredients. Work the wet ingredients into the dry ingredients with your hands.

Step 5: Continue working the mixture with your hands until it begins to resemble damp sand. Once the mixture will clump together in your hands, it is ready for the molds.

Step 6: Tightly pack the bath bomb mixture into the desired molds. Wait a minute or two.

Step 7: Pop the bath bombs carefully out of the mold and onto a flat surface covered with a plush, fluffy towel.

Step 8: Let the bath bombs dry completely for 24 to 48 hours.

Get Creative

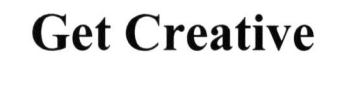

The fun thing with bath bombs is what also makes them so unique; you can alter each bath bomb to fit into a specific theme or cater to a specific person. You can add practically anything your heart desires into the bath bomb. Glitter, dried flower petals, another bath bomb (think 'Inception'), anything that can go into the tub can go into the bath bomb.

Adding Extras

If you're going to add extra things into the bath bomb that are not discussed in the recipe, you may be curious as to when you should add them. This all depends on what you are adding. If you are adding glitter, dried flowers, seeds, nuts and other dry items, you should add them to the dry ingredients before adding the liquid ingredients. Another option is line the bottom of the mold with the extra item. For example, place lavender buds, rosehips or glitter on the bottom of the mold before pressing the bath bomb mixture into the mold. This will keep the added items on the top of the bath bomb instead of dispersed throughout it.

The extras you add don't necessary have to be store bought either. You can grow your own herbs or go for a little natura walk to collect wildflowers to dry and add to your homemade bath bombs. Forging your own extra items to add to bath bombs make these wonderful and useful items even more budget-friendly.

Molds

You can also use just about anything as a mold, which increases the possibilities for your bath bombs. There are actual molds marketed for use in bath bomb making available at craft stores. However, there really is no need to spend the extra money when you can use the plastic candy molds, baking molds, muffin tins and a slew of other mold-like items you already have on hand. In fact, if you can pack the bath bomb mixture into it, you can probably use it as a mold.

Tips and Considerations

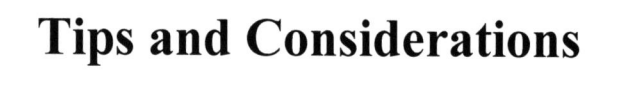

Recipes for bath bombs typically call for either water or witch hazel. While either or work perfectly fine for making your own bath bombs, witch hazel doesn't foam up as much when mixing the dry and liquid ingredients together. Because of this, witch hazel is usually preferred over water. However, not everyone keeps witch hazel on hand. For most crafters, the decision between witch hazel and water is purely based on preference.

If you are adding essential oils or coloring, add them to the liquid ingredients before adding the liquid ingredients to the dry ingredients. If you want bath bombs in different colors, simply divide the mixtures equally. For example, if you want bath bombs in blue, purple, pink and red, set out 8 separate bowls and equally divide the liquid mixture into 4 bowls and the dry mixture into 4 bowls. Add the blue coloring to 1 bowl filled with the liquid ingredients; add the purple coloring to another bowl filled with the liquid ingredients and so on and so forth. Remember to add one drop of coloring at a time, stirring after each drop until the desired color has been achieved.

I have found that if you lightly mist the bath bombs with witch hazel, it forms am exterior crust that helps to keep the bath bombs from cracking and falling apart. The process that has worked for me is to lightly mist with witch hazel after removing the bath bombs from the mold and let dry overnight. The next morning, turn the bath bombs over, mist the bottoms with the witch hazel and let dry for another day.

Bath bombs make the perfect gift for anyone, no matter what their age or hobbies; everyone needs a relaxing bath at some point to soothe tired and sore muscles or to relax a bit after a stressful day. And while the bath bombs themselves are the true gift, you don't just want to toss some in a plastic sandwich baggie and hand them out to people. You need to add some presentation to the gift. For example, you can purchase cute little Chinese take-out boxes that are perfect for filling with bath bombs. For a more rustic appearance, fill a miniature burlap sack with the bath bombs and tie close with a twin bow.

Conclusion

The age old saying, "If at first you don't succeed, try again" is something you should keep in mind while making bath bombs. When I first began making them, it was a lot of trial and error, with a few batches that were complete failures. I am so glad, however, that I kept at it because after about the third batch, I had the entire process down packed. I could probably even make bath bombs in my sleep!

No matter which recipe you try, remember to make the bath bombs your own. Put your unique touch into it. You are in complete control over what does and does not go into the bath bomb. And, above all else, have fun! If you're doing right, the bath bomb making process should be an enjoyable task that you look forward to completely.

Bath Salts

Introduction

I am a crafter at heart. And while many of my "projects" don't pane out as planned, there are a few that are so simple and fun to create that I just gotta keep making them. Bath salts is one of these do-it-yourself projects that really is a moneysaver, especially if you're like me and love to soak in a nice hot bath after a long hard day. And since I can be rather cheap at times, I just didn't want to continue to shell out $20 to $40 a month for high quality and boutique-style bath salts. Especially when I can make my own bath salts with my favorite fragrances at a fraction of what commercial bath salt blends costs. Seriously, you will spend only pennies on the dollar making your own blend, and if you take a lot of baths like I do, that savings will quickly rack up. Once you make your first batch and try it out yourself, you will continue to make more and more, altering the ingredients to match your style, mood and the even season! And since ingredients for homemade bath salts are pretty cheap and easy to come by, you can make special and one-of-a-kind gifts for all your friends and family.

Basic Ingredients

While bath salts are rather simple to make and can be altered to fit your needs, there is essentially one main ingredient that is required to successfully make your own bath salts; salt. Without salt, you could not get the therapeutic benefits the blend provides. In fact, you can simply use 2 cups of sea salt or Epsom salt in your bath and you will experience most of the benefits that commercial bath salts provide. But where's the fun in that? With that in mind, however, there are a few other ingredients that can increase the overall experience of the bath salt blend. For example, adding essential oils to the salt provides a bit of aromatherapy to your warm bath and can help ease tension, relieve stress and uplift your mood. You can also add a bit coloring for purely aesthetic reasons and dried or fresh herbs and flowers.

Most bath salts recipe will call for one of the following base-style ingredients:

- Epsom salts
- Sea salt
- Epsom salt and sea salt
- Epsom salt, clay and borax
- Epsom salt, baking soda and glycerin

If you don't have all the ingredients on hand at the moment, however, you can simply substitute the basic ingredients for one of the others listed above. For example, if the recipe calls for epsom salt, clay and borax, you can use sea salt in place of epsom salt. If you don't have clay and borax on hand, you can simply eliminate them from the recipe all together.

Borax? In Bath Salts?

Yes, some ingredients call for borax, but it's not the same type of borax that you use for cleaning. Using that kind of borax in your bathwater could be hazardous to your health. Instead, use borax powder from Moutain Rose. It doesn't contain the detergents and surfactants that are found in commercial borax powder. Instead, Mountain Rose borax powder acts as an emulsifier, buffering agent and natural preservative for your homemade bath salt blend.

Choosing the Right Ingredients

What type of salt you use for your bath salt base is an important factor to consider. Sea salt, however, is the most popular choice for bath salts. It has been used for centuries to help soften bath water and provide various benefits to the skin. Sea salt will vary in size and color depending on where the salt originated from. For example, salt from the Dead Sea has a clear or pure white color while salt from the Himalayas has a natural reddish or pinkish hue. These colors, however, can be altered with coloring if desired. A simple, inexpensive and effective alternative to sea salt is Epsom salts, which can be purchased at grocery stores, department stores, Dollar stores and online merchants. In fact, some bath salt recipes call for Epsom salt instead of sea salt. Some recipes even use a combination of Epsom salt and sea salt in the recipe. If the recipe you are using lists Sea salt as the base ingredient, you can substitute it with Epsom salt and still achieve the benefits of the bath salt blend. No matter what salt base you choose, never use table salt. It will do nothing but turn your bathwater salty.

Another option is "bath salts", which is readily available at craft stores both online and off. These commercial "bath salts" contain some form of salt and are marketed to crafters wanting to create their own homemade bath salt blend. While it may sound like a wonderful alternative to mixing your own salt based, commercial "bath salts" are usually more expensive and most crafters would rather save money without skimping on quality by purchasing the desired sea salt and/or Epsom salt in bulk.

Bath Salt Recipes

Lavender Bath Salts

Ingredients:

- 2 cups Epsom salts
- 25 milliliters water soluble lavender oil
- 25 milliliters sunflower or grapeseed oil
- Couple drops natural food coloring or soap coloring (optional)
- Few sprigs of lavender leaves and/or flowers

Directions:

Step 1: Pour the Epsom salts into a clean glass container that has a sealable lid.

Step 2: Drizzle the oils over the salt and stir thoroughly with a metal spoon.

Step 3: Add a few drops of the coloring and stir. Add a few more drops if necessary until you reach the desired shade.

Step 4: Rub the leaves of the lavender plant between your fingers. This will release the plant's essential oils and natural fragrance. Set the lavender leaves on the top of the bath salt mixture. Seal the glass jar with its lid until ready to use.

Tips and Considerations:

The lavender leaves are only to release its natural oils and fragrance into the bath salts. It is not for use in your bath water. The bath salts will need to be stirred before using since the oils sometimes settle at the bottom of the jar. When ready to use, stir the bath salts and then sprinkle them into the tub filled with warm water. You should let them dissolve completely before settling into the relaxing bath.

Eucalyptus and Vanilla Bath Salts

Ingredients:

- 1 cup Epsom salt
- 1/2 cup baking soda
- 3 drops eucalyptus essential oil
- 8 drops vanilla in jojoba oil
- Green food or soap coloring (optional)

Directions:

Step 1: Mix Epsom salt, essential oils and baking soda together in a large plastic sealable bag.

Step 2: Add one to two drops of green coloring to the mixture.

Step 3: Seal the bag closed.

Step 4: Massage the mixture on the outside of the plastic bag. If needed, add another drop of food coloring. Continue massaging the outside of the bag until the mixture is thoroughly combined.

Step 5: Pour the mixture into a glass container with a lid and store in a cool, dry location until ready to use.

Step 6: Use about 1 spoonful of bath salts for every bath.

Rosemary Bath Salts

Ingredients:

- 2 cups Epsom salt
- 2 tablespoons baking soda
- 2 drops of coloring (optional)
- 4 drops of rosemary essential oil

Directions:

Step 1: Mix the salt and baking soda in a clean mixing bowl.

Step 2: Drizzle the essential oil and food coloring over the dry ingredients and mix with a spoon until evenly distributed.

Step 3: Pour the mixture in a clean mason jar, secure the lid on the top of the jar and store in a cool, dry place.

Simply Aromatherapy Bath Salts

Ingredients:

- 300 grams salt crystals
- 4 to 5 drops of essential oil, such as peppermint, orange, lavender, rose, eucalyptus or ylang ylang.

Directions:

Step 1: Mix the salt crystals and desired essential oil together in a clean bowl.

Step 2: Transfer the mixture into a clean glass jar with a secure lid.

Step 3: Secure the lid on the glass jar and place the aromatherapy bath salts in a cool, dry place until ready to use.

Tips and Considerations:

When choosing essential oil for aromatherapy, consider what mood you are trying to achieve. Peppermint is uplifting and great for relieving muscle aches and tension headaches. Orange is a cleaning oil that helps dry skin while providing some relief from stress and colds. Calming lavender is wonderful for reducing headaches, providing relaxation and restoring emotional balance. Rose oil helps ease emotional stress and helps relieve dry skin. Eucalyptus clears blocked sinuses and helps ease the symptoms associated with colds, and ylang ylang relieves stress and helps calm anxious moods.

Rainbow Bath Salts

Ingredients:

- 2 pounds Epson salt
- Food coloring in various colors
- Small glass containers
- Lavender essential oil
- Ziploc bags
- Large mixing bowl

Directions:

Step 1: Separate the Epson salts equally into the Ziploc bags. Make sure to have 1 bag for each food color you are using.

Step 2: Place a drop or two of the food coloring in each bag. For example, blue food coloring in one bag, red food coloring in the second bag and so forth.

Step 3: Secure the bag closed and shake for several seconds until the ingredients are evenly dispersed.

Step 4: Add one to two drops of the lavender essential oil into the bags and mix again in the same manner as before.

Step 5: Pour a layer of one colored bath salts in the bottom of the glass container.

Step 6: Pour a second layer of the next colored bath salts on top of the first layer of bath salts. Continue in this manner until you have a jar filled with rainbow layered bath salts.

Rose Milk Bath Salts

Ingredients:

- 1 1/2 cup powdered milk (full fat or nonfat, either will work fine)
- 1/2 cup Epsom salts
- 1/4 cup dried rose petals (or more if so desired)
- Red food coloring
- Rose essential oil

Directions:

Step 1: Mix the Epsom salts and powdered milk together in a mixing bowl.

Step 2: Add 2 to 3 drops of the food coloring to the mixture and stir until you achieve a uniform pink hue.

Step 3: Add the rose petals and about 5 to 7 drops of rose essential oil to the mixture. Stir thoroughly with a wooden spoon,

Step 4: Pour the mixture into small sachets or glass bottles. You can hand them out as gifts or keep for yourself.

Step 6: Scoop the bath salts into cute little containers and give as Valentine's Day gifts to your friends and family.

Herbal Bath Salts

Ingredients:

- 2 cups Epsom Salt
- 1 cup Kosher salt
- Dried herbs
- Essential oils

Directions:

Step 1: Mix the salts together in a Ziploc bag.

Step 2: Add 8 to 12 drops of the desired essential oil. Lavender essential oil helps calms and relaxes you before bed, while mint energizes and boosts your moods.

Step 3: Squish the outside of the bag to mix and evenly distribute the oil.

Step 4: Pour the mixture into a re sealable container. Place a few tablespoons of dried herbs on the top. Alternatively, mix the dried herbs into the bath salt mixture if desired.

Step 5: Store the homemade bath salts in the container until ready to use. Add a few spoonfuls of the bath salts to the warm water and let dissolve before slipping into the tub.

Moisturizing Bath Salts

Ingredients:

- 2 cups Epsom Salt
- 1 cup Kosher salt
- 2 tablespoons of almond oil
- Essential oils

Directions:

Step 1: Mix Epsom salt and kosher salt together in a bowl.

Step 2: Drizzle the almond oil over the salts. Use your hands or a spoon to even disperse the almond oil through the salts.

Step 3: Transfer the mixture into a glass container and store in a cool, dry place.

Step 4: Use one to two spoonfuls of the moisturizing bath salts to your bath water when ready to use.

Mint Mojito Bath Salts

Ingredients:

- 2 cups sea salt, Epsom salt or kosher salt
- Fresh mint, diced finely
- Zest and juice of a lime
- Mint essential oil
- Green soap or food coloring (optional)

Directions:

Step 1: Stir the salt, mint, lime juice and lime zest together in a small bowl.

Step 2: Add 3 to 5 drops of essential oil. Stir the mixture once again.

Step 3: Add 1 or 2 drops of the green coloring to give the mixture a hint of green. You can omit this step if not coloring the bath salt mixture.

Step 4: Mix the all the ingredients together and store in an airtight container.

Step 5: When ready to use, add 1/2 cup of the homemade mint mojito bath salts to your warm bath.

Detoxifying Epsom Bath Salts

Ingredients:

- 2 cups Epsom salt
- 1 to 2 cups baking soda
- 1 tablespoon ground ginger

Directions:

Step 1: Plan for ahead for your detoxifying bath by not eating anything immediately before as well as immediately after the bath.

Step 2: Drink plenty of water before and after the bath to ensure your body stays hydrated.

Step 3: Mix the salt, baking soda and ginger together in a bowl.

Step 4: Fill the bathtub up with water, keeping the water as hot as your body can handle it. You want to promote sweating to help push the toxins out of your body.

Step 5: Pour the detoxifying bath salt mixture into the water and stir with your hand.

Step 6: Carefully get into the water, slipping down into it so it goes all the way to your neck. Let yourself soak for at least 20-minutes.

Step 7: When ready to get out of the tub, drain the water and carefully step out of the tub. You may feel a bit light headed or dizzy.

Step 8: Dry yourself off and continue to consume plenty of water.

Orange Dreamsicle Bath Salts

Ingredients:

- 3 cups Epsom salts
- Glycerin
- Orange Extract
- Vanilla Extract
- Red food coloring
- Yellow food coloring

Directions:

Step1: Measure 2 cups of Epsom salts and pour into a small mixing bowl.

Step 2: In a separate small bowl, mix together 2 teaspoons of glycerin and 1 teaspoon of orange extract.

Step 3: Add about 12 drops of red food coloring and 50 drops of yellow to the glycerin and extract mixture. Mix the ingredients together thoroughly. The color should be a pastel orange.

Step 4: Mix the colored mixture with the Epsom salts making sure the ingredients are evenly dispersed. This is the orange portion of the dreamsicle bath salts.

Step 5: Mix 1 teaspoon of glycerin and 1/2 teaspoon of vanilla extract together in a bowl. Add 1 cup of Epsom salt into the bowl and mix once again. This is the vanilla portion of the dreamsicle bath salts.

Step 6: Begin layering the two bath salts in clean glass containers. Old jelly jars work well. Start with the orange salts making a 2 to 3 inch layer, and then layer the vanilla salts on top. Continue in this manner until you have filled the jar. Screw the lid on the jar and store until ready to use.

Bath Salts for Back Pain

Ingredients:

- 2 cups Epsom salts
- 1 cup bi-carb soda
- 10 drops peppermint essential oil
- 5 drops rosemary essential oil
- 5 drops eucalyptus essential oil
- 5 drops cinnamon essential oil
- 5 drops lavender essential oil
- 1 tablespoon fresh rosemary sprigs
- 2 tablespoons dried lavender flowers

Directions:

Step 1: Combine the Epsom salts and bi-carb soda in a bowl.

Step 2: Drizzle the essential oils over the dry ingredients. Mix together with a spoon.

Step 3: Add the fresh rosemary sprigs and dried lavender flowers. Stir gently until the rosemary and lavender are well dispersed throughout the bath salt mixture.

Step 4: Store the homemade bath salts in an airtight container. When ready to use, add 1 cup of the mixture to your warm bath and soak for at least 15 minutes.

Lemon and Rosemary Bath Salts

Ingredients:

- 2 cups Epsom salts
- 1/2 cup baking soda
- 2 to 3 tablespoons fresh finely chopped rosemary
- 6 to 8 drops of lemon essential oil
- 2 to 3 tablespoons lemon zest (optional)

Directions:

Step 1: Combine the Epsom salt with baking soda in a bowl.

Step 2: Add 3 to 4 drops of the lemon essential oil. Stir thoroughly.

Step 3: Add the remaining 3 to 4 drops of essential oil and stir once again until the oil is evenly dispersed.

Step 4: Sprinkle the chopped rosemary and lemon zest over the mixture. Stir all the ingredients together with a large wooden or metal spoon.

Step 5: Transfer your homemade lemon and rosemary bath salts to an airtight storage container.

Grapefruit Bath Salts

Ingredients:

- 1 cup of sea salt
- Red food coloring
- Grapefruit essential oil

Directions:

Step 1: Pour the seal salt into a mixing bowl.

Step 2: Add a few drops of the red food coloring to the sea salt and stir with a metal spoon. If desired, add a bit more food coloring until the sea salt has a nice pinkish hue.

Step 3: Add about 4 drops of the grapefruit essential oil. Stir the mixture together with the spoon.

Step 4: Pour the homemade grapefruit bath salts into a mason jar. Secure the lid on the mason jar and set the bath salts in a cool, dry location until ready to use.

Simple Soothing Bath Salts

Ingredients:

- 1 cup Epsom salt
- 3 drops rose essential oil
- 3 drops jasmine essential oil

Directions:

Step 1: Combine the three ingredients above in a small bowl.

Step 2: Mix the ingredients together with a metal spoon.

Step 3: Pour the bath salts into an airtight container until ready to use.

Simple Re Relaxing Bath Salts

Ingredients:

- 1/4 cup Dead Sea salt
- 1/4 cup Epsom salt
- 2 cups Pacific Sea salt
- 20 drops lavender essential oil

Directions:

Step 1: Mix the Dead Sea salt, Epsom salt and Pacific Sea salt together in a clean mixing bowl.

Step 2: Drizzle the lavender essential oil over the salts.

Step 3: Work the essential oil into the salts with your fingers until well dispersed.

Step 4: Store the re relaxing bath salt mixture into a glass container with a lid until ready to use.

A Simple Feel Good Bath Salt Mixture

Ingredients:

- 2 cups Dead Sea salt
- 10 drops chamomile essential oil

Directions:

Step 1: Combine the Dead Sea salt and chamomile essential oil together in a small glass jar.

Step 2: Secure the lid on the glass jar and shake for several seconds until the salt and essential oil is thoroughly mixed.

Sensual Bath Salts

Ingredients:

- 1 cup Epsom Salt
- 4 cups Pacific Sea salt
- 5 drops lemon essential oil
- 10 drops ylang ylang essential oil

Directions:

Step 1: Combine the Epsom salt and Pacific Sea salt into a bowl.

Step 2: Pour the essential oils over the salts and stir with a spoon until the ingredients are well mixed.

Step 3: Transfer the sensual bath salts to a container with a lid and store in a dry place out of direct sunlight and away from direct heat.

Uplifting Bath Salts

Ingredients:

- 1 cup Pacific Sea salt
- 1 cup Dead Sea salt
- 20 drops rosemary essential oil

Directions:

Step 1: Pour the two types of sea salts into a mixing bowl. Stir with a wooden spoon.

Step 2: Drizzle the rosemary essential oil over the salt mixture. Stir the oil and salt together until the oil is well dispersed throughout the salts.

Step 3: Pour the bath salt mixture into a storage container until ready to use in your bathwater.

Refreshing Bath Salts

Ingredients:

- 1 cup Pacific Sea salt
- 1 cup Dead Sea salt
- 10 drops lavender essential oil
- 5 drops neroli essential oil

Directions:

Step 1: Mix the sea salts together in an airtight jar.

Step 2: Pour the lavender and neroli essential oil into the sea salts.

Step 3: Secure the lid on the airtight jar and shake for several seconds until the oil is thoroughly dispersed.

Step 4: When ready to use, add 1/2 to 1 cup of the bath salts per bath.

Energizing Bath Salts

Ingredients:

- 1 cup Pacific Sea salt
- 2 cups Epsom salt
- 10 drop rosemary essential oil
- 6 drops eucalyptus essential oil
- 15 drops peppermint essential oil

Directions:

Step 1: Combine the Pacific Sea salt and Epsom salt in a bowl.

Step 2: Drizzle the rosemary, eucalyptus and peppermint essential oil over the salts.

Step 3: Stir the ingredients with a metal spoon until well mixed.

Step 4: Transfer the ingredients into a glass jar with a lid.

Step 5: Add 1 cup of the mixture to warm bathwater. Stir the water and bath salts with your hand until the salts have dissolved.

Step 6: Store the remaining bath salts in a cool, dry location.

Extra Uplifting Bath Salts

Ingredients:

- 1 cups Pacific Sea salt
- 2 cups Epsom salt
- 6 drops neroli essential oil
- 3 drops lemon essential oil
- 8 drops orange essential oil
- 6 drops lavender essential oil

Directions:

Step 1: Combine all the ingredients in a medium-sized bowl.

Step 2: Pour the bath salt mixture in a glass airtight container.

Step 3: Use 1/2 to 1 cup of the mixture per bath. Store the remaining bath salts in a dry and cool area.

Bath Salts for Aches and Pains

Ingredients:

- 1 cup Epsom salt
- 1 cup Pacific Sea salt
- 1 cup Dead Sea salt
- 5 drops lavender essential oil

Directions:

Step 1: Combine the 4 ingredients in a mixing bowl. Make sure the essential oil is even dispersed throughout the salt mixture.

Step 2: Store the bath salts in an airtight container.

Tropical Bath Salts

Ingredients:

- 1 cup Pacific Sea salt
- 1 cup Epsom salt
- 4 drops lavender essential oil
- 2 drops eucalyptus essential oil

Directions:

Step 1: Mix the two salts together in a resealable container.

Step 2: Pour the two essential oils over the salts.

Step 3: Incorporate the essential oil into the salts by working the ingredients together with your hands.

Step 4: Once the mixture is well combine, secure the lid on the container and store until ready to use.

Bath Salts Tea Bag

Ingredients:

- 5 ounces sea salt
- 1 teaspoon of dried herbs, such as lavender, rose petals, chamomile, rosemary or mint
- Muslin tea bags measuring about 4 x 5.5 inches
- Yarn or string

Directions:

Step 1: Combine the salt and dried herbs together in a small bowl.

Step 2: Fill the muslin tea bags with the mixture. Secure the top of the bag close with the yarn or string, leaving about 12-inches of string left.

Step 3: When ready to use, tie the bath salt tea bag to the faucet and allow it to seep in your bathwater.

Step 4: Keep the tea bag in the water for as long as you are relaxing in the tub. When finished, toss the used tea bag in the trash.

Fruitylicious Bath Salts

Ingredients:

- 1 cup of Sea salt
- 2 drops apple fragrance
- 3 drops melon fragrance
- 1 drop lemon essential oil

Directions:

Step 1: Pour the salt in a small mixing bowl.

Step 2: Add the fragrance and essential oil over the salt, one drop at a time.

Step 3: Stir the mixture with a large spoon to evenly distribute the fragrance and oil through the salt blend.

Step 4: Pour the mixture in an airtight container. When ready to use, add a generous amount to your bathwater.

Dead Skin Removing Bath Salts

Ingredients:

- 1 cup Himalayan salt
- 2 cups Dead Sea salt
- 1 cup of raw oats, grinded down to a powder

Directions:

Step 1: Mix the ingredients together in a resealable container.

Step 2: Draw a warm bath.

Step 3: Pour a generous amount of the dead skin removing bath salts into the water and stir with your hand.

Step 4: Carefully slip in the tub and soak for at least 20 minutes.

The salts naturally cleanse your pores and help to lift toxins from your skin. This will leave your skin feeling soft and supple. The raw oats will also soothe and soften your skin and give it a healthy glow.

Autumn Orchard Bath Salts

Perfect for those cool autumn nights.

Ingredients:

- 1 cup of Sea salt
- 1 drop cinnamon fragrance
- 4 drops apple green fragrance

Directions:

Step 1: Pour the salt into a container.

Step 2: Add the cinnamon and apple green fragrance to the salt and stir well.

Step 3: Store the autumn orchard bath salts in a resealable container and place in an out-of-the-way location that is dry and cool.

Couple's Bath Salts

Ingredients:

- 1 cup sodium sesquicarbonate
- 1 cup Sherpa pink Himalayan salt, fine grain
- 2 drops peppermint essential oil
- 6 drops ylang ylang essential oil
- Handful of fresh rose petals

Directions:

Step1: Blend the sodium sesquicarbonate and salt together until well mixed.

Step 2: Incorporate the essential oils into the dry ingredients using a spoon or your hands to evenly distribute the ingredients.

Step 3: Draw a warm bath for you and your lover.

Step 4: Add the entire salt blend to the water. Use your hand to mix the warm bathwater and salt blend together.

Step 5: Sprinkle fresh rose petals on the top of the water. Light some candles, play some relaxing music and enjoy the bath with your love.

Easy To Make Bath Salt Blends in Bulk

Morning Orchard Bath Salts

Ingredients:

- 5 pounds Pacific Sea salt
- 50 drops apple green fragrance
- 25 drops green food coloring

Day at the Beach Bath Salts

Ingredients:

- 5 pounds Pacific Sea salt
- 60 drops ocean breeze fragrance
- 30 drops blue food coloring

Sweet Island Bath Salts

Ingredients:

- 5 pounds Himalayan salt
- 120 drops coconut fragrance

Pomegranate Splash Bath Salts

Ingredients:

- 5 pounds Pacific Sea salt

- 80 drops pomegranate fragrance
- 30 drops red food coloring

Directions:

Step 1: Choose one of the 4 bulk bath salts blend that you want to make.

Step 2: Put on a pair of latex gloves.

Step 3: Pour the salt in a large bowl.

Step 4: Add the food coloring to the salt, one drop at a time. Continuously blend the coloring with one gloved into the salt while adding the drops until you achieve the desired

Step 5: Add the fragrance to the blend, one drop at a time, while incorporating it into the bath salts with your gloved hand.

Step 6: Store the bath salt blend in a well-sealed container. Each recipe creates bath salts for about 25 baths.

Himalayan Bath Salt Blends

The Sunrise Bath

Perfect for early morning bathes when you just woke up and need a boost.

Ingredients:

- 1 cup Himalayan salt
- 5 drops tangerine essential oil
- 2 drops lime essential oil

The PMS Bath

When you're feeling the unpleasant affects from your monthly visitor, soak in a tub filled with warm water and this blend.

Ingredients:

- 1 cup Himalayan salt
- 3 drops peppermint essential oil
- 8 drops lavender essential oil

After-Hitting-the-Gym Blend

You've worked up quite a sweat at the gym and your muscles are tired and sore. Take a bath with this blend to provide a bit of relief and leave you feeling refreshed.

Ingredients:

- 1 cup Himalayan salt
- 4 drops peppermint essential oil
- 3 drops eucalyptus essential oil

The Time Machine Blend

When you need youthful skin, take a soak with this bath salt blend that will leave your skin radiant while reducing the appearance of wrinkles and fine lines.

Ingredients:

- 1 cup Himalayan salt
- 3 drops rosemary essential oil
- 6 drops geranium essential oil

Sleepy Time Bath Blend

If you're having problems sleeping at night, consider adding a nightly bath to your ready-for-bed routine.

Ingredients:

- 1 cup Himalayan salt
- 3 drops ylang ylang essential oil
- 8 drops lavender essential oil

Directions:

Step 1: Combine all the ingredients together in a bowl, making sure the essential oils are well dispersed throughout the salt.

Step 2: Prepare your bathwater and sprinkle the entire blend back and forth over the bathwater.

Step 3: Use your hand to stir the bath salt blend into the water. Enjoy your bath!

The Hangover Bath Salt Blend

When you awake the next morning after a night of indulgence, you often feel horrible. Achy, nausea and headaches will plague you for most of the day. Treating yourself to a detoxifying bath with this homemade salt blend will help relieve some of those hangover-like affects.

Ingredients:

- 1 cup Dead Sea salt or Epsom salt
- 2 drops juniper essential oil
- 5 drops grapefruit essential oil
- 3 drops lavender essential oil

Directions:

Step 1: Mix the salt and essential oils together in a bowl.

Step 2: Draw a bath with lukewarm water.

Step 3: Sprinkle the bath salt blend into the water. Use your hand to slowly swirl the water around until the bath salt blend is dissolved.

Step 4: Slowly slip into the tub. Lay a cool towel behind your head, to act as a cushion, and lay back.

Step 5: Fold a washcloth dampened with the lukewarm water and place it across the top of your forehead.

Step 6: Relax and soak for at least 20 minutes and don't forget to consume plenty of water throughout the day.

Bath Salt Blends for Men

Bath salts are not just for women and these manly bath salt blends prove that!

Neroli Bath Salt Blend

- 5 pounds minera Dead Sea salt
- 1 teaspoon neroli fragrance oil
- 20 drops yellow food coloring
- 20 drops red food coloring

Frankincense and Myrrh Bath Salt Blend

- 5 pounds minera Dead Sea salt
- 1 teaspoon frankincense and myrrh fragrance oil
- 25 drops yellow food coloring

Rosemary Bath Salt Blend

- 5 pounds Epsom salt
- 1 teaspoon rosemary essential oil
- 30 drops green food coloring

Direction for Each Recipe:

Step 1: Put on a pair of latex gloves.

Step 2: Pour the salt in a large bowl.

Step 3: Add the food coloring a few drops at a time while blending it into the salt with your hand.

Step 4: Add the essential oils and/or fragrance in the same manner as you did with the food coloring.

Step 5: Store the blend in an airtight container. Each recipe creates about 8 soaks in the tub.

Bath Salt Blends for Kids

You can create these blends for the kids in your family or have your little ones help create them with you!

Dragon Bath Salt Blend

- 5 pounds Pacific Sea salt
- 60 drops dragon's blood essential oil
- 10 drops yellow food coloring
- 30 drops red food coloring

Monster Mania Bath Salt Blend

- 5 pounds Pacific Sea salt
- 60 drops frankincense and myrrh essential oil
- 40 drops green food coloring

Sweet Meadow Bath Salt Blend

- 5 pounds Pacific Sea salt
- 120 drops lavender essential oil
- 30 drops violet food coloring

Princess Bath Salt Blend

- 5 pounds Pacific Sea salt
- 65 drops jasmine essential oil

- 30 drops red food coloring

Directions for Each Recipe:

Step 1: Put on latex gloves, this will prevent your hands from becoming stained with the food coloring.

Step 2: Pour the salt into a large bowl.

Step 3: Add the food coloring to the salt one drop at a time.

Step 4: Use your gloved hand to mix the food coloring into the salt.

Step 5: Add the essential oils to the colored salt one drop at a time.

Step 6: Use your gloved hand to mix the oils throughout the salt.

Step 7: Store the homemade bath salt blend in a well-sealed container. Each recipe should create enough for 25 baths.

Keep in mind, however, that children should always be surprised when creating bath salt blends. Furthermore, these bath salt blend recipes are not intended for babies.

Bath Salts as Gifts

Bath salts make a great economical homemade gift for any occasion. And since they are so versatile and easy to alter, you can make specific blends for your loved ones. For example, if Aunt Lois has back pain, whip her up a blend of the bath salts for back pain recipe. Or, if your sister-in-law Rachel has dry skin, make her the moisturizing bath salt blend.

Just remember that the presentation of the bath salts is almost as important as the bath salts themselves. You don't want to present your wonderful, homemade blend in a sandwich baggie, do you? Some people forgo the presentation because they think it isn't cost efficient. This simply isn't true. In fact, you can start saving small glass jars -- like jelly jars or baby food jars -- and fill them with your bath salt blend. Then, simply attach a sticker with the name of the bath salt blend on the top of side of the jar. You can purchase blank stickers at office supply centers and department stores. You can use these stickers in your home printer or you can simply write the bath salt blend name on them.

Another option is to fill mason jars with the bath salt blend and tie a ribbon or twin around the jar. You can attach a sticker to the jar if desired or tie a vintage-looking label to the ribbon or twin to create a more rustic look.

No matter how you decide to present your bath salt blend, remember to have fun and get creative!

Conclusion

While bath salts are extremely easy to create, you may find that you prefer more or less of the recommended ingredients. For example, some people prefer less essential oil or fragrance oil in their blend while others want a stronger scent. Altering the recipe is completely fine and most crafters will encourage you to experiment with the recipe. As long as you don't alter the amount of the basic ingredients (epsom salt, sea salt, etc), your homemade bath salt blend should still work as intended.

Body Butter

Introduction

Anyone who has ever tried body butter knows the luscious, skin-softening properties it possesses. Unfortunately, commercial body butter typically comes along with a high price tag and chemical ingredients that you wouldn't want to place on your skin. For those interested in a better option, make your own homemade body butter! Taking the do-it-yourself approach allows you complete control over the ingredients while still fitting into even the tightest budget.

Basic Ingredients and Tools

Even though the basic ingredients vary from one recipe to another, there are generally two main ingredients needed: liquid vegetable oil – such as olive oil, almond oil and sunflower oil – and solid vegetable fats, such as shea butter, palm oil or coconut oil. With this in mind, you can create your own body butter recipe that is unique to your needs and desires.

Essential oils are another ingredient that is commonly used in body butters but isn't necessarily required so they can usually be omitted if you don't have any on hand. Keep in mind, however, that essential oils provide various positive health effects that you will be missing out on if not added to the body butter.

As with the ingredients, there are a few tools you should have on hand when making body butter. Double boiler, stirring utensil, mixer and container is usually needed for the process. However, you can improvise on some of the tools. For example, if you don't have access to a double boiler then a glass bowl place on top of a pot of boiling water will work in a pinch. You can also simply use a pot or saucepan, making sure to stir constantly so the ingredients don't burn.

Another tool commonly used in when making your own body butter is an ice bath. An ice bath is essentially when a smaller bowl – typically filled with the ingredients you want to cool – is placed inside a larger bowl that is filled with ice. If you don't want to deal with the hassle of creating an ice bath, you can simple place the smaller bowl inside a refrigerator to cool.

Storing the Body Butter

It is best to store homemade body butter in amber or cobalt glass jars that are airtight. Clear glass jars will also work if they are kept out of direct sunlight and away from direct heat. Placing the jars in direct sunlight promotes oxidations, which ruins the body butter.

Many times, homemade body butters will begin to warm and melt, causing them to lose their whipped-like consistency. There is no need to panic and toss the body butter out if this occurs. Simply place it back into the refrigerator and re whip until it develops the desired constancy once again.

Shelf Life of Body Butter

Since most homemade body butters don't contain a preservative, their shelf life is less than that of commercial body butters. However, trying to pinpoint the exact shelf life is difficult since each body butter recipe contains varying ingredients. A good general rule of thumb, however, is to keep the body butter unrefrigerated for up to 2 months. Placing the body butter in the fridge will increase its lifespan but causes it to become hard. Instead, keep the body butter in a cool room and use within 2 months.

Body Butter Recipes

Whipped Body Butter

Ingredients:

- ½ cup mango or cocoa butter
- ½ cup shea butter
- ½ cup coconut oil
- ½ cup light olive, jajoba or almond oil
- 10 to 30 drops of essential oil (optional)

Directions:

Step 1: Combine the butters and oils together in a double boiler.

Step 2: Place the double boiler over medium heat and stir the ingredients constantly until they are completely melted.

Sep 3: Remove the melted mixture from heat and let cool for several minutes.

Step 4: Place the mixture in the refrigerator to cool for about an hour or until it begins to harden but is still a bit soft.

Step 5: Remove the mixture from the fridge and whip with a hand mixer until fluffy, which is usually about 10 minutes or so.

Step 6: Place the mixture back into the fridge for 10 to 15 minutes to allow it to set.

Step 7: Transfer your homemade whipped body butter to a glass jar with a lid until ready to use.

White Chocolate Whipped Body Butter

Ingredients:

- 1 cup cocoa butter
- 1 cup coconut oil

Directions:

Step 1: Add the cocoa butter and coconut oil into a saucepan.

Step 2: Place the saucepan on the stove set on low to medium heat.

Step 3: Stir the butter and oil with a wooden spoon continuously until the two ingredients are completely melted.

Step 4: Transfer the melted mixture into a clean container. Place inside a refrigerator until it begins to firm and becomes hardened.

Step 5: Remove the hardened body butter from the refrigerator. Use a hand mixer to whip the butter into a fluffy and light consistency.

Step 6: Store the white chocolate whipped body butter in a cool place.

Wild Rose Body Butter

Ingredients:

- 7 ounces shea, avocado or mango butter
- 2 ounces sunflower oil
- ½ ounce rosehip seed oil
- 8 drops rose absolute
- 10 drops geranium rose essential oil
- ½ teaspoon rose clay
- 2 teaspoons tapioca starch

Directions:

Step 1: Add the butter to a clean mixing bowl. Use a hand mixer to mix the butter. Start with the lowest speed and gradually increase the speed until the butter has a fluffy and light consistency.

Step 2: Add the sunflower oil, rosehip oil, geranium rose essential oil, rose clay and rose absolute.

Step 3: Mix the added ingredients into the butter with the mixer. Start at the lowest speed, gradually increasing it until the butter is light and fluffy. When the consistency resembles buttercream frosting, stop mixing.

Step 4: Spoon the homemade body butter into jars and secure the cap tightly. This recipe should fill about eight 2-ounce sized jars.

Soothing Lavender and Mint Body Butter

Ingredients:

- ¼ cup extra virgin coconut oil
- 3.4 cup Grade A unrefined shea butter
- 2 tablespoons calendula petals, dried
- 2 tablespoons marshmallow root, dried and cut up
- 8 drops lavender essential oil
- 8 drops peppermint essential oil

Directions:

Step 1: Preheat the oven to 200-degrees.

Step 2: Melt the coconut oil and shea butter together on the stove over low heat in an oven-safe pan. Stir in the petals and marshmallow root.

Step 3: Turn the oven off and immediately place the mixture-filled, oven-safe pan inside the oven.

Step 4: Let the mixture steep inside the oven for at least four hours.

Step 5: Remove the pan from the oven. If the mixture has solidified, simply warm it up over low heat on the stove until it melts again.

Step 6: Strain the herbs out of the oil using cheesecloth or a mesh strainer. Dispose of the herbs and place the oil in a mixing bowl.

Step 7: Place the oil-filled mixing bowl into the refrigerator until it becomes firm not solid. This typically takes a few hours.

Step 8: When the oil is firm, remove it the mixing bowl from the fridge and whip the oil with a hand mixer for about 30seconds.

Step 9: Use a spatula to scrape the sides and bottom of the bowl when the body butter starts to stick so you can thoroughly whip all the butter with the mixer.

Step 10: Add the essential oils to the body butter.

Step 11: Use the hand mixer to whip the essential oils into the body butter.

Step 12: Continue to whip the body butter until it starts to turn while and peaks form.

Step 13: Store the body butter in an airtight container until ready to use.

Mint Chocolate Body Butter

Ingredients:

- ½ cup cocoa butter, grated
- ½ cup shea or mango butter
- ½ cup coconut oil
- ½ cup mild olive or jojoba oil
- 1 to 2 teaspoons peppermint essential oil
- 2 tablespoons pure cocoa powder (if you want a version that isn't a bronzer and is more "white chocolate", use non-GMO cornstarch or arrowroot powder instead.)
- 2 teaspoons vitamin E (optional)

Directions:

Step 1: Place a small bowl – that can hold at least 5 cups of liquid -- in the middle of a larger bowl. Fill the larger bowl with ice.

Step 2: In a double boiler, melt the butters over low simmering heat.

Step 3: Add the coconut oil and continue melting until the ingredients are liquefied.

Sep 4: Remove the mixture from the stove.

Step 5: Gradually add the cocoa powder to the olive or jojoba oil.

Step 6: Add the cocoa powder and oil mixture to the melted butter/oil mixture, stirring together until well mixed.

Step 7: Transfer the mixture to the small bowl surrounded by ice and resting in the middle of the larger bowl. Let the mixture cool for 10 minutes.

Step 8: Once the mixture has cooled, add the essential oil and Vitamin E (if desired) and stir for several seconds.

Step 9: Remove the small bowl from the larger ice-filled bowl.

Step 10: Use a mixer to whip the mixture on medium to high speeds until stiff peaks begin to form. If the mixture isn't thickening, place the small bowl back into the larger ice-filled bowl and continue whipping.

Step 11: When the mixture has the consistency similar to buttercream frosting, transfer to container and store until ready to use.

Magnesium Body Butter

Ingredients:

- ½ cup magnesium flakes
- 3 tablespoons boiling water
- ¼ cup coconut oil, unrefined
- 2 tablespoons beeswax pastilles
- 3 tablespoons shea butter

Directions:

Step 1: Mix the magnesium flakes and boiling water in a small container. Stir until the flakes are well dissolved. You should be left with a thick liquid. Set the container aside for the moment to cool.

Step 2: Fill a small pan with about 1 inch of water and place on the stove.

Step 3: Sit a quart-sized mason jar in the middle of the small pan on the stove.

Step 4: Add the oil, beeswax and shea butter into the mason jar.

Step 5: Turn the stove on medium heat and allow the ingredients to melt, stirring with a wooden spoon.

Step 6: Remove the mason jar from the pan when the ingredients have completely melted. Let it cool to room temperature.

Step 7: Pour the contents of the mason jar into a blender. Blend the ingredients on medium speed.

Step 8: Add the magnesium mixture one drop at a time into the blender while still continuously blending the ingredients. Continue in this manner until all of the magnesium mixture has been added.

Step 9: Place the blender jar into the refrigerator for about 15 minutes and then re-blend until the consistency is that of body butter.

Step 10: Store the magnesium body butter in a cool location for up to two months.

Mint Infused Coconut Body Butter

Ingredients:

- 2 tablespoons shea butter
- 1 tablespoon mint-infused coconut oil
- 1 tablespoon olive oil
- Rose petals, dried
- Rosemary, fresh
- 1 capsule Vitamin E
- 7 drops lime essential oil
- 7 drops lavender essential oil

Directions:

Step 1: Melt the shea butter and coconut oil together in a pan over low to medium heat. Stir consistently to prevent the butter and oil from burning.

Step 2: Add the vegetable oil, dried rose petals and fresh rosemary to the melted mixture. Stir together and then simmer on low for 20 minutes.

Step 3: Let the mixture cool for a few minutes and then strain the herbs from the liquid.

Step 4: Open the vitamin E capsule and dump the contents inside the cooled liquid. Add the essential oils.

Step 5: Use a hand mixer to whip the ingredients together. Continue whipping until the body butter develops the right consistency.

Step 6: Store the butter in an airtight container.

3-Ingredient Cocoa Body Butter

Ingredients:

- 1.75 ounces cocoa butter
- 1.75 ounces wheat germ oil
- ½ teaspoon vitamin E oil (optional)

Directions:

Step 1: Place the cocoa butter in a double boiler over medium heat and melt.

Step 2: Remove the melted butter from heat and allow to cool for a few minutes.

Step 3: Once cool, add the wheat germ oil and vitamin E to the cocoa butter, stirring thoroughly for several seconds.

Step 4: Place the mixture into a fridge for about 5 to 10 minutes.

Step 5: After the allotted time, remove the mixture from the fridge and whip the ingredients with a hand mixture until the mixture develops a creamy consistency.

Step 6: Transfer the homemade body butter into an airtight container until you are ready to use.

Coconut Oil and Honey Body Butter

Ingredients:

- 1 ½ cups coconut oil
- 3 tablespoons honey
- 2 tablespoons grapefruit zests (any other citrus zests can be used)

Directions:

Step 1: Combine the coconut oil, honey and zest in a mixing bowl.

Step 2: Whip the ingredients together with a hand mixer until the consistency is creamy and a bit fluffy.

Step 3: Scoop the mixture into an airtight container or glass jar.

Simple Mango Body Butter

Ingredients:

- 3.5 ounces mango butter
- 2 tablespoons coconut oil
- 1 tablespoon beeswax
- 4 tablespoons kukui nut oil
- 3 tablespoons distilled water

Directions:

Step 1: Use a double boiler to melt the mango butter, coconut oil and beeswax together.

Step 2: Remove the melted mixture from the heat and allow to cool for several minutes.

Step 3: Add the kukui nut oil and distilled water to the mixture and stir until well mixed.

Step 4: Use a hand mixer to whip the body butter into a creamy consistency.

Step 5: Scoop out the body butter and store in an airtight container.

Coconut and Mango Body Butter

Ingredients:

- 30 grams coconut oil
- 30 grams mango butter
- 20 grams shea butter
- 30 drops mango essential oil

Directions:

Step 1: Place the coconut oil and shea butter into a pan. Heat the two ingredients on low to medium until the melt and become a liquid.

Step 2: Add the mango butter and then stir the ingredients slowly with a wooden spoon.

Step 3: Turn off the heat and let the mixture cool for 10 to 20 minutes, but don't let is set completely.

Step 4: Add the mango essential oil to the mixture and stir once again with the wooden spoon.

Step 5: Use a hand mixer to whip the ingredients until they are light and fluffy.

Step 6: Store the body butter in an airtight container.

3-Ingredient Shea Body Butter

Ingredients:

- 2.5 ounces shea butter
- 1 ounce macadamia nut oil
- 10 drops grapefruit essential oil

Directions:

Step 1: Melt the shea butter in a double boiler. When completely melted, remove from heat and let cool for several minutes.

Step 2: Add the macadamia nut oil and grapefruit essential oil and stir for several seconds until well mixed.

Step 3: Place the mixture into the refrigerator for about 6 minutes.

Step 4: Remove the cooled mixture from the fridge and use a hand mixer to whip the ingredients into a creamy consistency.

Step 5: Place the body butter in a jar and store in an cool, dry location.

Extreme Moisturizing Body Butter for Dry and Damaged Skin

Ingredients:

- 3.5 ounces shea butter
- 2.5 ounces coconut oil
- 1.75 ounces cocoa butter
- 1.75 ounces mango butter
- 1.75 macadamia oil
- 1.25 ounces avocado oil
- 1.25 jojoba oil
- 1.25 almond oil

Directions:

Step 1: Melt the butters and the coconut oil together in a double boiler.

Step 2: Remove the mixture from the heat when the ingredients are completely melted. Allow to cool for several minutes.

Step 3: Add the macadamia oil, avocado oil, jojoba oil and almond oil to the melted mixture. Stir thoroughly with a wooden spoon.

Step 4: Place the mixture back into the fridge for about 8 minutes.

Step 5: Remove the mixture from the fridge and whip with a hand mixer until you achieve a creamy consistency.

Step 6: Transfer the body butter into an airtight container until ready to use.

Hand Softener Body Butter

Ingredients:

- 2.5 ounces illipe butter
- 1 ounce almond oil
- 10 drops of essential oil (optional)

Directions:

Step 1: In a double boiler, melt the illipe butter.

Step 2: Remove the melted butter from the heat and allow to cool for several minutes.

Step 3: Add the almond oil and essential oils to the melted butter and stir until all ingredients are well mixed.

Step 4: Place the mixture in the refrigerator for 4 minutes.

Step 5: Remove the mixture from the fridge and whip it into a creamy consistency with a hand mixer.

Step 6: Transfer the mixture into a container.

Step 7: Use as a hand softening mask by massage the body butter into your hands before bed and then wearing cotton gloves while sleeping.

Cocoa and Hemp Body Butter

Ingredients:

- 3 tablespoons coconut oil
- 1 tablespoon beeswax
- 1 tablespoon castor oil
- 1 tablespoon sunflower oil
- 1 tablespoon hemp seed oil
- 1 tablespoon honey
- 10 drops essential oil (optional)

Directions:

Step 1: In a double boiler, melt the coconut oil and beeswax.

Step 2: Remove the melted oil and wax from heat and let cool for a few minutes.

Step 3: Stir in the rest of the oils and the honey.

Step 4: Use a hand mixer to whip the ingredients until they develop a creamy consistency.

Step 5: Pour the body butter into the container you are storing it in.

Aloe, Coconut and Lavender Body Butter

Ingredients:

- 4 tablespoons coconut oil
- 1 ½ tablespoons olive oil
- 2 tablespoons beeswax
- 1 teaspoon honey
- 3 tablespoons aloe vera gel
- 2 teaspoons lanolin
- 10 drops lavender essential oil
- 1 vitamin E capsule

Directions:

Step 1: Heat the oils, beeswax and honey over medium heat in a double boiler.

Step 2: In a separate saucepan, heat the aloe over medium heat until melted.

Step 3: Add the melted aloe into the melted mixture in the double boiler. Stir thoroughly.

Step 4: Add the lanolin to the mixture and stir together.

Step 5: Once all the ingredients are melted, remove from heat.

Step 6: Break open the vitamin E capsule and dump its contents into the mixture.

Step 7: Add the essential oil.

Step 8: Use a hand mixer to whip the ingredients until they are smooth.

Step 9: Store in airtight glass jars.

Peppermint Tallow Whipped Body Butter

Ingredients:

- 1 cup shea butter
- ½ cup tallow
- ½ cup jojoba oil
- 1 teaspoon peppermint essential oil
- 2 teaspoons vitamin E oil

Directions:

Step 1: Slowly heat the shea butter and tallow until the two ingredients are melted.

Step 2: Remove the butter and tallow from heat. Add the jojoba oil and stir with a wooden spoon.

Step 3: Let the ingredients chill in an ice bath for about 5 minutes.

Step 4: Stir in the peppermint essential oil and vitamin E oil.

Step 5: let the mixture chill in the ice bath a bit longer until it is completely chilled.

Step 6: Whip the homemade body butter with a hand mixer until stiff peaks begin to form.

Step 7: Transfer the body butter into airtight glass jars. Store the jars out of direct sunlight.

Vanilla Bean Body Butter

Ingredients:

- 1 cup raw cocoa butter
- ½ cup sweet almond oil
- ½ cup coconut oil
- 1 vanilla bean

Directions:

Step 1: Melt the butter and coconut oil over low heat. Remove the mixture from heat and let cool for for about 30 minutes.

Step 2: Grind the vanilla bean in a food processor or coffee grinder.

Step 3: Mix the sweet almond oil and bits of vanilla bean into the butter and oil mixture.

Step 4: Chill the mixture in the fridge for about 20 minutes. You want the oils to begin to solidify without completely hardening.

Step 5: Use an electric mixture to whip the mixture into a butter-like consistency.

Step 6: Store the body butter in glass jars.

Information: This recipe makes about 3 cups of whipped body butter.

Anti-Bacterial Body Butter

Ingredients:

- ½ cup coconut oil
- 6 tablespoons cocoa butter
- 2 tablespoons jojoba oil
- Few drops of Progest E (optional)
- 15 to 20 drops tea tree oil

Directions:

Step 1: Place the cocoa butter in an oven-safe glass container. Place the container in an oven set on low temperature for several minutes until the cocoa butter melts but doesn't become too hot.

Step 2: Remove the container from the oven and add the coconut oil and jojoba oil Stir the ingredients together until well combined.

Step 3: Set the mixture on the kitchen counter where it won't be disturbed for several hours or overnight. You want the mixture to start to solidify.

Step 4: Whip the solidified mixture for 6 to 10 minutes with a hand mixture. Stop and scrape the mixture off the sides if necessary.

Step 5: Add the tea tree oil to the body butter and whip once again with the hand mixture.

Step 6: Store the antibacterial body butter until ready to use.

Key Lime Whipped Coconut Oil Body Butter

Ingredients:

- ½ cup coconut oil
- 1 tablespoon olive oil (macadamia nut oil or castor oil can be used instead)
- 2 tablespoons aloe vera gel
- 20 drops lemon essential oil
- 20 drops lime essential oil

Directions:

Step 1: Place all the ingredients together in a mixing bowl.

Step 2: Set an electric mixer with a wire whisk attachment on high and whip the ingredients together for 3 to 7 minutes until you achieve an airy, light consistency.

Step 3: Scoop the whipped body butter into airtight glass jars. Store the homemade body butter in a cool, dry place.

Whipped Peppermint Body Butter

Ingredients:

- ½ cup coconut oil
- ½ cup cocoa butter
- ½ cup shea butter
- ½ cup sweet almond oil
- 1 teaspoon vitamin E oil
- 2 to 4 drops peppermint essential oil

Directions:

Step 1: Fill a medium-sized pot with the coconut oil, cocoa butter and shea butter. Set the pot on the stove and melt under low heat making sure to stir constantly until the ingredients are completely melted.

Step 2: Remove the pot from the heat.

Step 3: Mix the sweet almond oil, vitamin E and peppermint essential oils into the melted ingredients.

Step 4: Allow the mixture to chill in the fridge for about an hour or two. The mixture will be ready when it is firm but not completely solidified.

Step 5: Whip the ingredients with a hand mixer or stand mixer until you achieve a whipped yet smooth consistency.

Step 6: Fill glass jars with the body butter and store at room temperature out of direct sunlight and away from direct heat.

Lavender Body Butter

Ingredients:

- 4 tablespoons coconut oil
- 1.5 tablespoons olive oil
- 2 tablespoons beeswax
- 1 teaspoon honey
- 3 tablespoons aloe vera gel
- 2 teaspoons lanolin
- 10 drops lavender essential oil
- 1 vitamin E capsule

Directions:

Step 1: Place a double boiler on medium heat. Add the oils, beeswax and honey to the double boiler and melt.

Step 2: Heat the aloe in a second double boiler until melted.

Step 3: Add the aloe to the oils, beeswax and honey. Stir thoroughly for several seconds.

Step 4: Add the lanolin and stir once again.

Step 5: Remove the mixture from the heat.

Step 6: Open the vitamin E capsule and pour the contents into the mixture.

Step 7: With a hand mixer, whip the contents until it achieves the consistency of body butter.

Step 8: Let the butter cool before storing it in airtight containers.

Rosemary Mint Body Butter

Ingredients:

- 45 grams cocoa butter
- 90 grams shea butter
- 45 grams kukui nut oil
- 20 drops spearmint essential oil
- 10 drops rosemary essential oil

Directions:

Step 1: Add the cocoa butter and shea butter into a glass dish.

Step 2: Drizzle the kukui nut oil over top the two butters.

Step 3: Set the glass bowl on top of a pan filled with simmering water.

Step 4: Let the ingredients melt over the simmering water. Stir constantly while the ingredients are melting.

Step 5: Remove the glass dish from heat and let cool to room temperature.

Step 6: Let the mixture cool for about 10 minutes before transferring it to the freezer to cool for an addition 20 minutes.

Step 7: Remove the mixture from the freezer. Whisk the mixture with a hand mixer for about 5 minutes before placing it back into the freezer for 15 to 20 minutes.

Step 8: Remove the mixture from the freezer yet again and whisk with the mixer until you achieve a fluffy, airy consistency. If necessary, return the mixture to the freezer for an addition 15 minutes before whisking again.

Step 9: Fill the airtight container with the body butter and place in a cool location until you are ready to use.

Coconut & Rose Body Butter

Ingredients:

- 60 grams coconut oil
- 10 grams jojoba oil
- 1 milliliter alkanet infused oil
- 3 grams cornstarch
- 10 drops rose essential oil

Directions:

Step 1: Place the coconut oil, jojoba oil, alkanet infused oil and cornstarch in a glass bowl.

Step 2: Place a pan filled with water on the stove and bring the water to a boil. Turn the heat down so the water stays at a simmer.

Step 3: Place the glass bowl filled with the first 4 ingredients on top of the pan filled with simmering water.

Step 4: Let the ingredients melt, mixing them all together with a whisk. Remove the mixture from the heat and let cool to room temperature.

Step 5: Add the essential oil to the mixture once it cools to room temperature.

Step 6: Whisk all the ingredients together until you achieve a light and fluffy consistency.

Step 7: Enjoy! Store the leftover body butter in an airtight glass jar.

Cinnamon Body Butter for Cellulite

Ingredients:

- 100 grams coconut oil
- 50 grams cocoa butter
- 50 grams shea butter
- 30 drops cinnamon oil
- Cinnamon Stick

Directions:

Step 1: Warm the cocoa butter and shea butter on the stove with low or medium heat. Stir constantly until the two ingredients have melted.

Step 2: Slowly add the coconut oil to the mixture and stir for about a minute.

Step 3: Remove the ingredients from the heat and let cool for 10 to 20 minutes.

Step 4: Once cooled, immediately add the cinnamon oil.

Step 5: Use a mixer to whip the ingredients into a fluffy, light consistency.

Step 6: Scoop the body butter into small glass, airtight jars.

Step 7: Break the cinnamon stick into small pieces. Stick a piece of the cinnamon stick into each jar of body butter.

Step 8: Secure the lid on the jars. Give the jars of homemade body butter to your friends and family! But don't forget to keep some for yourself!

Edible Chocolate Body Butter

Ingredients:

- ¾ cup coconut oil, melted
- 1/3 cup clear agave nectar
- ½ tablespoon vanilla powder
- ¼ cup cacao powder (add a bit more if you want a thicker texture)

Optional Ingredients

- ½ teaspoon cistanche (an herb that promotes sexual prowess)
- 1 teaspoon maca (known to balance hormones and strengthens libidos)
- 1 to 2 drops rose essential oil
- ½ teaspoon powdered lavender flowers

Directions:

Step 1: Add all the desired ingredients into a food processor.

Step 2: Blend the ingredients until they are well incorporated.

Step 3: Transfer the mixture into a glass jar.

Step 4: Store the mixture either in the fridge or in a cool room until ready to use.

Coffee Body Butter Foot Cream

Ingredients:

- 0.7 ounces white beeswax
- 3.1 ounce coffee butter
- 2.4 ounces sunflower oil
- 1.2 ounces stearic acid
- 1 ounce emulsifying wax
- 15.6 ounces distilled water
- 5 milliliters dark rick chocolate fragrance oil
- 5 milliliters peppermint 2nd distillation essential oil
- 0.2 ounce optiphen

Directions:

Step 1: Using a microwave, melt the emulsifying wax, beeswax, stearic acid, coffee butter and sunflower oil together in a heat-safe container.

Step 2: In a separate heat-safe container, heat the distilled water to around 150 to 155 degrees.

Step 3: The temperature of the oil mixture must be within 5 to 10 degrees of the water's temperature. If it is not, stick the oil mixture back into the microwave for a few seconds.

Step 4: Pour the oil mixture carefully into the water and blend continuously for 3 minutes.

Step 5: Add the optiphen, chocolate fragrance oil and peppermint essential oil to the mixture, stirring until well blended. The temperature of the mixture cannot be above 176 degrees when adding the preservative optiphen or it will render it ineffective. Keep this in mind when adding it to the mixture.

Step 6: Microwave the mixture once again for a few minutes until it is warm.

Step 7: Immediately pour the mixture into glass jars. Let the jars sit overnight before placing the lid on them.

Step 8: Use a spoon to whip the mixture up inside the jars. Secure the jar closed with its lid and place in a cool room.

Dreamy Lemon Cream Body Butter

Ingredients:

- 6 tablespoons coconut oil
- ¼ cup cacao butter
- 1 tablespoon vitamin E oil
- ¼ teaspoon lemon essential oil

Directions:

Step 1: Combine the coconut oil and cacao butter in a saucepan and melt over low heat.

Step 2: Remove the saucepan from heat. Add the essential oil and vitamin E oil, stirring with a spoon.

Step 3: Let the mixture cool for a few hours at room temperature.

Step 4: Transfer the body butter to an airtight container.

Super Glowy Body Butter

Ingredients:

- 2 cups organic coconut oil, extra virgin and raw
- 7 ounces shea butter
- 1 drop tea tree oil
- Essential oil of your choice (such as lavender, peppermint or jasmine)

Directions:

Step 1: Melt the coconut oil and shea butter together in a double boiler.

Step 2: Remove the mixture from heat.

Step 3: Mix the tea tree oil and essential oil to the mixture. Blend for about 1 minute.

Step 4: Allow the mixture to cool and begin to solidify. This will take several hours at room temperature. You can speed the process up by placing the mixture in the fridge.

Step 5: Once the mixture has solidified, whip it into a light and fluffy consistency with a hand mixer.

Step 6: Scoop the body butter into airtight glass jars.

Black Raspberry and Vanilla Body Butter

Ingredients:

- 156 grams cocoa butter
- 155 grams shea butter
- 24 grams grapeseed oil
- 65 grams apricot kernel oil
- 4 grams vitamin E oil
- 10 grams black raspberry vanilla fragrance oil

Directions:

Step 1: Melt the butters, grapeseed oil and apricot kernel oil together in a double boiler. Heat until the ingredients are completely melted and well mixed.

Step 2: Remove the mixture from the heat. Add the vitamin E oil and fragrance oil. Stir for several minutes.

Step 3: Transfer the mixture to a clean mixing bowl. Place the missing bowl inside a separate, larger bowl that is filled with ice.

Step 4: Let the mixture cool in the ice bath for 20 minutes.

Step 5: Remove the mixture from the ice bath. Use a hand mixer to whip the ingredients for several minutes. Place the mixture back into the ice bath for an additional 20 minutes.

Step 6: Repeat Step 5 until the mixture develops a consistency of whipped butter.

Step 8: Scoop the body butter into airtight containers until ready to use.

The Simplest Body Butter

Ingredients:

- 1 cup cocoa butter
- ½ cup coconut oil
- ½ cup sweet almond oil

Directions:

Step 1: Melt the butter and oil together in a double boiler or saucepan.

Step 2: Transfer the melted mixture to mixing bowl. Add the sweet almond oil and blend.

Step 3: Place the mixture in the freezer for about 20 minutes until it has become solid but not hard.

Step 4: Use an electric whisk to whip the mixture into a fluffy white cloud.

Step 5: Spoon the mixture into a clean container until ready to slather it on.

The Wonderful Body Butter Recipe

Ingredients:

- 1 cup organic coconut oil
- 1 teaspoon vitamin E oil
- 3 drops pure vanilla essential oil

Directions:

Step 1: Place all the ingredients in a large mixing bowl.

Step 2: Use an electric mixer to whip the ingredients into a fluffy, soft consistency.

Step 3: Transfer the body butter to several small jars or one larger airtight glass container.

Sacred Frankincense Body Butter

Ingredients:

- ½ cup coconut oil, virgin and organic
- ½ cup shea butter
- ½ cup mango butter
- 1 ounce cocoa butter, raw and organic
- 1 teaspoon vitamin E oil
- 30 drops sacred frankincense essential oil

Directions:

Step 1: Combine the shea butter, mango butter and cocoa butter together in a double boiler. Let the three ingredients melt.

Step 2: Pour the melted butters into a clean mixing bowl.

Step 3: Stir the coconut oil into the melted butters.

Step 4: Let the mixture cool on the counter top for about 45 minutes.

Step 5: Stir the vitamin E oil and frankincense essential oil into the mixture.

Step 6: Cover the mixing bowl and place inside the fridge for about 40 minutes. You want the mixture to begin to solidify but not become too hard.

Step 7: Whip the mixture with a hand mixer until fluffy peaks form.

Step 8: Scoop the body butter into mason jars and store in a cool location.

Ultra Moisturizing Body Butter

Ingredients:

- ½ cup shea butter
- ½ cup mango butter
- ½ cup coconut oil
- ½ cup liquid oil, such as almond, sunflower, olive or grapeseed
- 2 tablespoon arrowroot powder
- 1 teaspoon vitamin E oil

Directions:

Step 1: Melt the butters and coconut oil together in a double boiler.

Step 2: Remove the mixture from the heat and let cool for about 20 minutes.

Step 3: Place the cooled mixture into an ice bath.

Step 4: While the mixture is cooling in an ice bath, mix the liquid oil, vitamin E oil and arrowroot powder together in a separate bowl.

Step 5: When the mixture in the ice bath begins to harden with a small pool of liquid on the top, add the oil/arrowroot concoction and whisk with a hand mixer.

Step 6: Continue whisking until it develops the consistency of creamy whipped butter. If the mixture isn't solid enough to whip, return it to the ice bath for an additional 20 minutes.

Step 7: Transfer the body butter to an airtight container to store until needed.

Scrumptious Body Butter

Ingredients:

- 3 ounces shea butter
- 2 ounces mango butter
- 1 ounce coconut oil
- 3 ounces grapeseed oil
- ½ ounce beeswax
- 2 ounces distilled water
- 2 ounces aloe vera gel
- Essential oils of your choice (optional)

Directions:

Step 1: Melt the butters, oils and wax together in a double boiler, stirring occasionally.

Step 2: Once melted, pour the mixture into a blender and let cool.

Step 3: Pour the distilled water and aloe vera gel in a small bowl and let come to room temperature.

Step 4: When the butter, oil and wax mixture has cooled completely, turn on the blender and slowly add the water and aloe vera gel. If necessary, scrape down the sides of the blender.

Step 5: Once completely blended, add your desired essential oils and continue to blend. Skip this step if you are not using essential oils.

Step 6: Once the body butter achieves the desired consistency, transfer to glass jars. The body butter can be stored at room temperature in a cool room or in a fridge.

Shea and Coconut Body Butter

Ingredients:

- ½ cup shea butter
- ¼ cup coconut oil
- ¼ cup almond or olive oil
- 10 to 15 drops essential oil

Directions:

Step 1: Mix all the ingredients together in a double boiler and melt over medium heat.

Step 2: Once the ingredients are melted and well blended, pour into a mixing bowl and let cool in a fridge for about 30 to 60 minutes.

Step 3: Remove the bowl from the fridge.

Step 4: Whip the mixture with a hand mixer for about 10 minutes, or until the mixture begins to resemble whipped cream.

Step 5: Scoop the body butter into a storage jar.

Sugar Cookie Body Butter

Ingredients:

- 100 grams cocoa butter
- 100 grams mango butter
- 100 grams shea butter
- 48 grams argan oil
- 52 grams fractionated coconut oil
- 4 grams vitamin E oil
- 10 grams sugar cookie fragrance oil

Directions:

Step 1: Melt the butters, argan oil and coconut oil together in a double boiler, stirring continuously.

Step 2: Remove the melted mixture from heat and add the vitamin E and sugar cookie fragrance oil. Stir the ingredients together with a stainless steel spoon.

Step 3: Transfer the mixture into a clean mixing bowl. Place the bowl in an ice bath or set inside the fridge to cool. The mixture will become thicker as it cools.

Step 4: Every 20 minutes, use a hand mixer to whip the body butter for several minutes before returning it to the ice bath or fridge.

Step 5: Repeat Step 4 until the mixture resembles whipped butter.

Step 6: Spoon the mixture into the jars and enjoy!

Honey Kissed Body Butter

Ingredients:

- ¾ cup cocoa butter
- ¾ cup shea butter
- 2 tablespoons jojoba or apricot kernel oil
- ¼ teaspoon vitamin E oil
- 1 tablespoon honey powder

Directions:

Step 1: Melt the cocoa and shea butter together in a double boiler.

Step 2: Remove the mixture from heat and stir in the remaining ingredients with a metal spoon.

Step 3: Let the mixture sit out on your kitchen counter for several hours to cool.

Step 4: Use a hand mixer to whip the mixture until it resembles whipped cream.

Step 5: Store the mixture in an airtight container.

Sparkling Citrus Mango Body Butter

Ingredients:

- 2/3 cup shea butter
- 1/3 cup mango butter
- 1 teaspoon jojoba oil
- 3 teaspoons grapeseed oil
- ¼ teaspoon vitamin E oil
- 10 drops bergamot essential oil
- 8 drops palmarose essential oil
- 8 drops lemongrass essential oil
- 2 drops cypress essential oil
- 1 drop rose geranium essential oil
- 1 teaspoon cornstarch
- Cosmetic mica (gives it a glittery appearance)

Directions:

Step 1: Melt the shea and mango butter together in a double boiler.

Step 2: Remove the melted butters from heat. Stir in the remaining ingredients.

Step 3: Let the body butter cool for several hours. To speed up the cooling process, sit the mixture inside the fridge.

Step 4: With a hand mixer, whip the mixture for several minutes until it develops the consistency similar to whipped cream. If necessary, return the mixture to the fridge to cool longer before continuing to whip.

Step 5: Use a metal spoon to scoop the mixture into glass jars. Store the body butter-filled jars in a cool location out of direct sunlight.

Lavender Spice Body Butter

Ingredients:

- 1/4 cup cocoa butter
- 1 cup shea butter
- 2 tablespoons Kukui or Sweet Almond oil
- 1 tablespoon jojoba oil
- 1 tablespoon rosehip oil
- 1/4 teaspoon vitamin E
- 1 teaspoon cornstarch
- 20 drops lavender essential oil
- 4 drops patchouli essential oil
- 4 drops sandalwood essential oil
- 2 drops cedarwood essential oil

Directions:

Step 1: In a double boiler, melt the cocoa and shea butter. Once completely melted, remove from heat.

Step 2: Add the remaining ingredients and stir with a metal spoon.

Step 3: Let the mixture sit for several hours until completely cooled and beginning to harden.

Step 4: Grab your hand mixer and whip the mixture until it has a consistency that is light and fluffy, similar to whipped cream.

Step 5: Spoon the mixture into small glass jars.

Lavender Flower Body Butter

Ingredients:

- 1/4 cup cocoa butter
- 1 cup shea butter
- 2 tablespoons Kukui or Sweet Almond oil
- 1 tablespoon jojoba oil
- 1 tablespoon rosehip oil
- 1/4 teaspoon vitamin E
- 1 teaspoon cornstarch
- 20 drops lavender essential oil
- 5 drops frankincense essential oil
- 2 drops palmarosa essential oil
- 2 drops rose germanium essential oil

Directions:

Step 1: In a double boiler, melt the cocoa and shea butter. Once completely melted, remove from heat.

Step 2: Add the remaining ingredients to the melted butters and stir with a metal spoon.

Step 3: Allow the mixture sit for several hours until completely cooled and beginning to harden.

Step 4: With a hand mixer, whip the mixture until it has a consistency that is light and fluffy. The body butter should have the consistency of whipped cream.

Step 5: Spoon the mixture into small glass jars and share with friends and family!

Body Butter To Die For

Ingredients:

- 2 tablespoons shea butter
- 1 tablespoon mint infused coconut oil
- 1 tablespoon olive oil
- Dried rose petals
- Fresh rosemary
- 1 vitamin E capsule
- 7 drops lime essential oil
- 7 drops lavender essential oil

Directions:

Step 1: Melt the shea butter and coconut oil together in a double boiler.

Step 2: Add the vegetable oil and stir with a metal spoon.

Step 3: Add the dried rose petals and fresh rosemary. Heat the mixture on low for about 20 minutes. Remove the mixture from heat.

Step 4: Strain the rose petals and rosemary from the liquid. Let the mixture cool until it reaches room temperature.

Step 5: Open the vitamin E capsule and dump the contents into the mixture. Add the essential oils and stir with a metal spoon.

Step 6: Whip the mixture for 5 to 10 minutes until it has a light and airy consistency. If the mixture isn't developing the right consistency, place it in the fridge to cool for a bit longer.

Step 7: Use a spatula to scoop the body butter into an airtight jar.

Manly Body Butter

Ingredients:

- ½ cup olive oil, extra virgin
- ¼ cup coconut oil, extra virgin
- ½ cup water
- 1 tablespoon vitamin E oil
- 1 tablespoon vitamin D oil
- 1 teaspoon tea tree oil
- 2 ounces beeswax

Directions:

Step 1: Combine the olive oil, coconut oil, water and beeswax in a small pot.

Step 2: Heat on low to medium until the ingredients are melted.

Step 3: Pour the melted mixture into a mixing bowl.

Step 4: Use an electric mixer to beat the mixture for several minutes.

Step 5: Add the vitamin E, vitamin D and tea tree oil to the mixture. Mix once again for several minutes.

Step 6: Place the mixture in the fridge for a couple of minutes before removing it and beating it once again for 3 to 4 minutes.

Step 7: Repeat Step 6 until the mixture has the consistency of whipped cream.

Step 8: Spoon the mixture into a glass jar and use when needed.

White Chocolate and Peppermint Body Butter

Ingredients:

- 1/4 cup cocoa butter
- 1/4 cup coconut oil, virgin or refined
- 1/8 cup avocado oil
- 1 teaspoon red raspberry seed oil
- 10-15 drops of peppermint essential oil

Directions:

Step 1: Melt the cocoa butter, coconut oil and avocado oil together in a double boiler. Use a whisk to gently stir the ingredients together while melting.

Step 2: Remove the mixture from heat and allow to cool for several minutes.

Step 3: Add the raspberry seed oil to the mixture and stir with the whisk until well incorporated.

Step 4: Place the mixture in the fridge for about an hour. You want the mixture to cool and the liquid to begin setting up, but still soft enough for you to whip.

Step 5: Remove the mixture from the fridge and add the peppermint essential oil.

Step 6: With a hand mixer, whip the body butter for several minutes until it resembles whipped cream.

Step 7: Transfer the mixture to glass storage jars.

Sweet Citrus and Vanilla Body Butter

Ingredients:

- ¼ cup kokum butter
- ¼ cup coconut oil, virgin or refined
- 1/8 cup jojoba or avocado oil
- 1 teaspoon red raspberry seed oil
- 25 to 30 drops vanilla essential oil
- 15 drops tangerine essential oil
- 15 drops sweet orange essential oil
- 10 drops lemon essential oil

Directions:

Step 1: In a double boiler, melt the kokum butter, coconut oil and jojoba or avocado oil. Use a whisk to gently stir the ingredients together while melting.

Step 2: Once the ingredients are melted but not too hot, remove the mixture from heat and allow to cool for a few minutes.

Step 3: Add the raspberry seed oil to the mixture and stir with the whisk until well incorporated.

Step 4: Place the mixture in the fridge for about an hour. You want the mixture to cool and the liquid to begin setting up, but still soft enough for you to whip.

Step 5: Remove the mixture from the fridge and add the vanilla, tangerine, orange and lemon essential oil. Mix together with a metal spoon.

Step 6: Use a hand mixer to whip the body butter until it resembles whipped cream. Transfer the mixture to glass storage jars.

Lavender and Vanilla Body Butter

Ingredients:

- ¼ cup mango butter
- ¼ cup coconut oil, virgin or refined
- 1/8 cup avocado oil
- 1 teaspoon red raspberry seed oil
- 15 to 20 drops lavender essential oil
- 25 to 30 drops vanilla essential oil
- 4 to 8 drops carrot seed essential oil

Directions:

Step 1: In a double boiler, melt the cocoa butter, coconut oil and avocado oil. Use a whisk to gently stir the ingredients together while melting.

Step 2: Once the ingredients are melted but not too hot, remove the mixture from heat and allow to cool for several minutes.

Step 3: Add the raspberry seed oil to the mixture and stir with the whisk until well incorporated.

Step 4: Place the mixture in the fridge for about an hour. You want the mixture to cool and the liquid to begin setting up, but still soft enough for you to whip.

Step 5: Remove the mixture from the fridge and add the lavender, vanilla and carrot seed essential oil.

Step 6: With a hand mixer, whip the body butter for several minutes until it resembles whipped cream.

Step 7: Transfer the mixture to glass storage jars.

2-Ingredient Coconut and Vanilla Body Butter

Ingredients:

- 16 ounces coconut oil
- Vanilla extract

Directions:

Step 1: Place the coconut oil into a mixing bowl.

Step 2: Set a stand or hand mixer on high and mix the coconut oil for about 2 to 4 minutes. Make sure to stop the mixer every so often and scrap the coconut oil stuck on the sides down.

Step 3: Add a cap full of vanilla extract to the oil and continue mixing for an additional 4 to 5 minutes. The mixture should have a fluffy consistency.

Step 4: Scoop the body butter out and into small glass jars.

Belly Butter for Pregnancy

Ingredients:

- 1/2 cup organic mango
- 1/4 cup organic shea butter
- 1/4 cup organic cocoa butter
- 1/2 cup organic coconut oil
- 1/4 cup avocado oil
- 1/4 cup rosehip seed oil
- 2 tablespoons arrowroot powder or organic cornstarch
- 1 teaspoon vitamin E oil
- 1 teaspoon neroli essential oil
- 1 teaspoon lavender essential oil
- 1/2 teaspoon frankincense essential oil

Directions:

Step 1: In a double boiler, melt the mango, shea and cocoa butter. Add the coconut oil and stir with a wire whisk.

Step 2: Remove the melted butter and oil mixture from the heat.

Step 3: In a separate bowl, mix the arrowroot and avocado oil, stirring until the powder is completely dissolved.

Step 4: Stir the arrowroot and oil mixture into the melted mixture. Add the rosehip seed oil and stir again.

Step 5: Transfer the mixture to a mixing bowl and let cool in the fridge for a few hours.

Step 6: Remove the mixing bowl from the fridge and add the essential oils and vitamin E oil.

Step 7: With a hand mixer, whip the mixture on medium to high speed until it resembles a light and fluffy whipped cream.

Step 8: Transfer the belly butter to airtight jars.

Step 9: When ready to use, rub a small amount of the butter into your belly to help restore moisture to your skin.

Body Butter for Eczema

Ingredients:

- 2.5 ounces raw organic cocoa butter, shaved
- 3.5 ounces unrefined raw organic shea butter
- 3 tablespoons organic apricot oil
- 1 teaspoon vanilla extract
- ½ teaspoon vegetable glycerin

Directions:

Step 1: Place the shaved cocoa butter in a double boiler and melt on low to medium heat.

Step 2: Place the shea butter into a food processor. Pulse the food processor a few times to warm and loosen up the shea butter.

Step 3: Drizzle the melted cocoa butter over the shea butter. Add the apricot oil, vanilla and glycerin.

Step 4: Blend all the ingredients in the food processor until the mixture has a creamy and velvety texture.

Step 5: Scoop the mixture out of the food processor and into airtight glass jars.

Coconut and Plum Body Butter

Ingredients:

- 2 ounces coconut cream oil, virgin and organic
- 2 ounces cocoa butter, ultra refined
- 1 ounce plum kernel oil
- 1/2 ounce carnauba wax
- 1 ½ teaspoons plum jojoba wax beads

Directions:

Step 1: Melt the cocoa butter, coconut oil and waxes together in a double boiler over medium heat.

Step 2: Once melted, add the plum kernel oil and stir with a metal spoon.

Step 3: Remove the mixture from heat and place in an ice bath.

Step 4: After several minutes, use an electric mixer to whip the body butter into a light and airy consistency.

Step 5: When the body butter reaches the correct consistency – resembling frosting or whipped cream – spoon it into airtight containers.

Body Butter Bars

Ingredients:

- 1 cup shea butter
- 1cup cocoa butter
- 1cup sweet almond oil
- 2 cups beeswax pellets
- ½ cup jojoba oil
- ½ cupvirgin coconut oil
- ¼ teaspoon rose absolute
- ¼ teaspoon cocoa absolute

Directions:

Step 1: In a double boiler, heat the shea butter, cocoa oil, almond oil and beeswax together until just melted.

Step 2: Remove from heat and let cool for 2 minutes.

Step 3: Add the jojoba oil, coconut oil, rose absolute and cocoa absolute to the mixture and stir with a metal spoon.

Step 4: Pour the mixture into soap molds or a baking pan.

Step 5: Let the body butter cool and harden before removing them from the molds and wrapping in plastic wrap or storing in an airtight container.

Tips and Considerations

Homemade body butter makes a thoughtful and well-loved gift for any occasion. In fact, some brides-to-be are making their own unique body butter to hand out as favors at their wedding. If you decide to give the gift of homemade body butter, remember to dress it up a bit. For an impressive presentation, scoop the homemade body butter into a piping bag – typically used for icing cakes and cookies – and pipe the body butter neatly into the gift containers. If you don't have piping bags on hand, you can make one by snipping the tip of the corner off a baggie and using that as a makeshift piping bag. Also consider, printing out a custom label that can be achieved to the top of the jar's lid. These labels can be printed with various pictures or words to fit your needs. For example, you can print labels that merely say 'Merry Christmas", or make them a bit more personalized with 'From Amanda's Kitchen'. Once the body butter is inside the jar, tie a cute ribbon around the jar to finalize the presentation.

If making the body butter for children, avoid certain essential oils – such as peppermint – and instead use something a bit more gentle like lavender essential oil, which is typically recommended for children.

Conclusion

When making homemade body butter, the most important thing to remember is to have fun! Experiment with the many different essential oils that you can add. The essential oil itself provides various health benefits that can improve your overall well-being. For example, lavender has both calming and anti-bacterial properties, while clove can clear nasal decongestion and rose can improve the look of your skin. Mix and match ingredients to create your very own recipe that you can pass down for generations to come.

Body Scrubs

Introduction

A popular staple at spas, body scrubs can be simple or complex, depending on what ingredients you use. Nevertheless, they are all beneficial in their own way. Not only do they exfoliate skin, but some body scrubs can also ease joint pain, relax tired muscles, increase circulation and rejuvenate skin. In fact, those are just a few of the potential benefits that homemade body scrubs can provide. If you haven't already, you should make body scrubs a must-have in your shower routine.

But why purchase costly and unimpressive commercial body scrubs when you can simply make your own?

I like to consider myself a craftster, always looking for things to create for myself, my family and my friends. So when I came across a recipe for homemade body scrub several years ago, I knew I had to try it as soon as possible. At the time, I was buying commercial body scrubs that were too expensive and just rather blah. And they never smelled as nice as they claimed. The strawberry shortcake body scrub that I purchased from a major retailer smelled less like strawberry shortcake and more like an overly sweetened chemical. I had paid in the double digits for something that I ultimately didn't use and just tossed in the trash. It was maddening! Therefore, I was extremely excited to try my hands at creating my own body scrub. I got the ingredients together, skimmed through the recipe and got started.

I'm not going to lie, my first batch was less than perfect and I almost gave up on the idea. But I pushed forward. With the fail batch in the garbage, I started once again and quickly realized that this batch was a bit easier to work with. The ingredients were meshing well together and the body scrub started to take form. I had gotten the hang of it.

Since then, I have regularly made body scrubs not just for myself, but also for my loved ones. About three times a year, I gather my ingredients in bulk and begin making batch after batch of homemade body scrubs.

Start Your Journey Here

Before you can begin your journey into the fun and exciting world of homemade body scrubs, you must first familiarize yourself with the basic ingredients, tools and process required for creating your own body scrubs.

Arm Yourself: The Tools and Ingredients Needed to Make your Body Scrubs a Hit

There are essentially three main ingredients that are required for a successful body scrub: exfoliant, carrier oil and essential oil. There are many options within these three categories to choose from. Therefore, it's not uncommon for those new to the whole homemade body scrub scene to feel a bit intimidated by all the choices. Thankfully, the following information will help get you acquainted with the basic ingredients of body scrubs, so you're not going into the process blind.

Exfoliant

While sugar and salt are the two most common ingredients used as an exfoliant in homemade scrubs (more about those later), there is actually various other ingredients that work well as an exfoliant. Ground coffee and oatmeal are two popular alternatives to sugar and salt.

Ground coffee not only gives the body scrub a pleasant aroma, but also provides benefits to the skin. Furthermore, the caffeine naturally found in coffee is a vasoconstrictor. In layman's terms, caffeine causes the blood vessels to constrict, which helps to reduce – albeit temporarily – rosacea and varicose veins.

Oatmeal is an extremely gentle exfoliant. In fact, it is the gentlest exfoliant for body scrubs. Oatmeal is also an emollient, which means it hydrates and softens the skin. For decades, people have used oatmeal as a home remedy for itchy, dry skin. Unlike the other exfoliants, water can be used as a carrier oil for oatmeal body scrubs.

Flax meal, almond meal, ground nutshells, buckwheat, wheat bran, cornmeal and rice bran also work well as an exfoliant for your homemade body scrubs.

Carrier Oil

Carrier oil – sometimes called base oil – is essentially what holds the ingredients of the body scrub together while acting as a moisturizer for the skin. As with exfoliants, there are a wide array of carrier oils to choose from, many with different benefits to consider. Most recipes – expect for those that tackle dry skin – generally call for a carrier oil that has a thin consistency, which means it washes off the skin easily and doesn't leave a greasy residue behind.

- Olive oil is probably the easiest carrier oil to get your hands on, and it's rather inexpensive to boot. If you use olive oil for your homemade body scrub, make sure to choose the lightest grade available, so the oil's natural scent doesn't cover up the smell of any essential oils you are using in the recipe. Olive oil has a shelf life of about a year.
- Sunflower oil has a thin consistency, is practically odorless and can penetrate the skin. In addition, sunflower oil is typically less expensive than other carrier oils and has about a 12-month shelf life.

- Grape seed oil is a very thin oil that absorbs easily and has a faint, sweet aroma. Its shelf life is typically between 6 and 12 months.
- Sweet almond oil has a nutty, somewhat sweet fragrance. This medium consistency oil absorbs into the skin quickly and has a shelf life of up to 12 months.
- Jojoba oil is known for its moisturizing capabilities without leaving behind a greasy residue on your skin. It works great for sensitive skin and has a stable shelf life that increases when added to other carrier oils.
- Hazelnut oil is a nutty-smelling carrier oil with a thin consistency that will leave a film on your skin. Its shelf is around 12 months.
- Vitamin E oil is a light, soft option for body scrubs. Unfortunately, it is rather expensive, and some DIYers choose to use a bit of this oil with another carrier oil to make it last longer.

- Kukui Oil and its thin consistency absorb well into the skin. It has a sweet yet light nutty aroma and shelf life of about 12-months.
- Macadamia nut oil is a thick oil that will leave an oily film behind. This nutty-smelling oil has a shelf life of 12-months and works best for dry skin.

Keep in mind that those are only some of the possible carrier oils you can use for your homemade body scrub.

Essential Oils

While essential oils can often be eliminated from the recipe, they do provide many benefits that make their presence invaluable to the body scrub. Essential oils – which are derived from and contain the compounds of plants – not only give the body scrub a pleasant aroma, they are also beneficial for your health.

Sweet or Salty: The Difference between Sugar Body Scrubs and Salt Body Scrubs

Sugar and salt have a similar appearance and can be hard to distinguish by looks alone. When they are used in a body scrub, however, you can quickly tell the difference between the two. Both contain coarse grains that work as an all-natural exfoliator to help remove the dead cells that accumulate on the top layer of your skin. Once the dead cells are removed, your skin will appear rejuvenated, fresh and glowing. However, both sugar and salt have their own specific benefits that you should consider when choosing your ingredients.

Salt for Homemade Body Scrubs

Salt is more abrasive than its sweeter counterpart is and works best for troubled areas, such as elbows and heels. Salt also absorbs oil, which makes it ideal for skin plagued with acne. Salt naturally has anti-viral and anti-bacterial properties, and a body scrub containing salt can help improve circulation when rubbed over your skin. Since salt is more abrasive than sugar, it works better to remove the layer of dead cells on rough, dry skin. Another thing to consider is that unlike sugar scrubs, homemade scrubs made with salt are not sticky and usually fall off while rubbing into the skin. This can lead to excessive waste of the scrub.

Sugar for Homemade Body Scrubs

While sugar is still an exfoliator, it is more gentle than salt. This is due to the sugar granules being round, which means it doesn't cut into the skin. Its gentle nature makes sugar the better ingredient for people with sensitive skin. Furthermore, sugar body scrub can be safely used on the face. The granules in the sugar scrubs dissolve easily in hot water, but don't contain the mineral benefits that you receive with salt scrubs. Sugar scrubs, however, are less drying and suitable for all skin conditions and types. Sugar also naturally contains glycolic acid, which helps to protect your skin from harmful toxins and is vitally important for skin health. Glycolic acid also can moisturize and condition. Sugar scrubs are stickier and softer than salt scrubs and will remain on your skin while applying. This allows the oils to stay put longer, giving them time to work their magic.

So, which ingredient should I use for my homemade sugar scrub?

It all really depends on your specific situation. Armed with the information discussed above, you should be able to choose the right ingredient for your needs. For example, if Aunt Deloris complains about the bottom of her feet being rough, use salt in her batch and save the sugar for your family members who have sensitive skin.

The Body Scrub Recipes

For the Newbie: Simple and Easy Body Scrub Recipes for Beginners

The following body scrubs are perfect for those just starting out in the wonderful world of homemade body scrubs. Not only are these recipes easy to create, but they also use ingredients that most people keep on hand or can easily acquire.

Basic Sugar Scrub

Ingredients:

- ¼ cup olive oil
- ¼ cup granulated white sugar
- 2 to 3 drops essential oil (optional)

Directions:

Step 1: Pour the white sugar and olive oil in a small mixing bowl.

Step 2: With a metal spoon, mix the two ingredients together. Add the essential oil if desired and mix once again.

Step 3: Transfer the sugar scrub to an airtight container. It will keep for about a month.

Basic Salt Scrub

Ingredients:

- ¼ cup olive oil
- ½ cup sea salt
- 2 to 3 drops essential oil (optional)

Directions:

Step 1: Add all the ingredients together in a mixing bowl.

Step 2: Stir together with a metal spoon for several seconds until the oil and salt are well mixed.

Step 3: Scoop the salt scrub into an airtight container. Use within a month.

The Manicure in a Jar

Ingredients:

- ¼ cup brown sugar
- ¼ cup olive oil
- 2 to 3 drops lavender essential oil
- 3 drops vanilla extract

Directions:

Step 1: Dump the brown sugar in a mixing bowl. Use a metal spoon to break up any lumps in the sugar.

Step 2: Add the olive oil, lavender essential oil and vanilla extract. Mix thoroughly with a spoon.

Step 3: Transfer the mixture to an airtight glass jar. Store in a cool, dry location and use within a month.

Simple Banana Sugar Scrub

Ingredients:

- 1 banana, ripe and starting to turn brown
- 3 tablespoons granulated sugar
- ¼ teaspoon pure vanilla extract (optional)

Directions':

Step 1: Pour the sugar into a bowl.

Step 2: Place the banana on top of the sugar and mash the two ingredients together.

Step 3: Add the vanilla extract and mix until well combined.

Step 4: Use the banana sugar scrub on your body before taking a shower or bath, massaging it into your skin. Rinse the scrub off your body and pat dry with a towel.

Simple Chocolate Body Scrub

Ingredients:

- 1 cup coconut oil
- ½ cup brown sugar
- ¼ cup cocoa powder

Directions:

Step 1: Combine the coconut oil, brown sugar and cocoa powder together in a mixing bowl.

Step 2: Transfer the mixture into airtight glass container until ready to use.

Ultimate Sea Salt Scrub

Ingredients:

- ½ cup baby oil
- 1 cup course sea salt

Directions:

Step 1: Mix the two ingredients together in an airtight storage container.

Step 2: Place a cover over the container and let sit for 24 hours.

Step 3: Stir the body scrub with a spoon and store in a cool, dark place until ready to use.

Gardener's Sugar Hand Scrub

Ingredients:

- Dawn dish soap
- White sugar
- 2 tablespoons olive oil

Directions:

Step 1: Fill the container – such as a mason jar – about ¾ full of sugar.

Step 2: Fill the remaining ¼ of the jar with the dawn dish soap.

Step 3: Let the dish soap soak for a minute or two before stirring the two ingredients together with a spoon.

Step 4: Add a bit more sugar and the olive oil to top it off. Stir with a spoon.

Step 5: Use whenever your hands are dirty from yard and gardening work.

Mind, Body and Soul: Homemade Body Scrubs for Health and Well Being

The following body scrub recipes are perfect for improving your overall health and well being. They can be used as part of your regular health or skin care regiment or whenever you deem necessary.

Relaxation Body Scrub with Lavender

Lavender is a fragrant flowering herb that has long been used to promote relaxation and help sleep. Studies have also shown that lavender can help relieve anxiety and headaches while soothing muscles and promoting good circulation.

Ingredients:

- I cup sea salt
- ½ cup of olive oil
- 5 to 7 drops of lavender essential oil
- 1 tablespoon dried lavender flowers (optional)

Directions:

Step 1: Mix the salt, oil and essential oil together in a small bowl.

Step 2: Add the dried flowers. Use a metal spoon to fold the dried lavender flowers into the mixture.

Step 3: Spoon the mixture into an airtight jar.

Hydration and Softening Body Scrub with Sweet Almond Oil

Sweet almonds naturally contain vitamin E and a high amount of oleic acid, which is an omega-9 fatty acid. And while some people think sweet almond oil is a moisturizer, it is, in fact, an emollient that softens skin without hydrating it. With that being said, sweet almond oil is also a humectant, which helps to prevent moisture loss. Sweet almond oil helps relieve itchy, dry and flaky skin and will easily absorb into your skin without the unpleasant, greasy residue. This recipe is suitable for all skin types.

Ingredients:

- I cup sugar
- ½ cup of sweet almond oil

Directions:

Step 1: Mix the sugar and sweet almond oil together in a small bowl with a metal spoon.

Step 2: Transfer the mixture into an airtight jar.

Anti-Aging Rosehip Body Scrub

Rosehip oil contains a high amount of concentrated vitamin A, which helps increase elastin and collagen in the skin and makes your skin supple. Vitamin E – which helps to fight skin aging – is also found in rosehip oil. All these beneficial aspects of rosehip oil mean that this essential oil can promote the growth of healthy skin cells.

Ingredients:

- I cup sugar
- ½ cup of coconut or olive oil
- 5 to 7 drops of rosehip essential oil
- 1 tablespoon dried rose flowers (optional)

Directions:

Step 1: Combine the sugar, oil and rosehip together in a metal bowl.

Step 2: Add the dried rose flowers, using a metal spoon to fold the dried flowers into the mixture.

Step 3: Spoon the mixture into an airtight jar.

Step 4: Lightly rub the homemade rosehip body scrub directly on age spots, wrinkles and dry areas of your skin.

Detoxifying and Exfoliating Dead Sea Salt Body Scrub

Dead Sea salt has long been used to treat a wide array of skin conditions including psoriasis. It is also an effective exfoliator that softens and detoxifies the skin. Studies have shown that Dead Sea salt helps promote healthy cell regeneration and improve blood circulation.

Ingredients:

- I cup Dead Sea salt
- ½ cup of olive oil, coconut oil or sweet almond oil
- 5 to 7 drops of the essential oil of your choice (optional)

Directions:

Step 1: Mix the salt and oils together in a small mixing oil. Make sure all the ingredients are incorporated into each other.

Step 2: Transfer the mixture into an airtight jar and store in a cool location.

Customizable Daily Face Scrub

This face scrub – which can be stored for up to 2 months -- can be used daily and can be customized to fit your specific skin type.

Ingredients:

- 1 teaspoon oats, finely ground
- 1 teaspoon almond meal, ground
- 1 teaspoon powdered milk
- ½ to 1 teaspoon water

Add for Oil Skin:

- 2 tablespoons fine sea salt
- 5 drops rosemary essential oil
- 2 tablespoons dried peppermint, finely ground

Add for Dry Skin:

- 2 tablespoons full fat powdered milk
- 5 drops chamomile essential oil
- 2 tablespoons calendula, finely ground

Add for Combination Skin:

- 2 tablespoons cornmeal
- 5 drops lavender essential oil
- 2 tablespoons dried chamomile, finely ground

Directions:

Step 1: Mix the oats, almond meal, powdered milk and water together in a small mixing bowl.

Step 2: Add the extra ingredients if desired for your specific skin type. Stir together with a metal spoon.

Step 3: Store the face scrub in an airtight container and use every morning to keep your skin clean and fresh.

Body Scrub for Extremely Sensitive Skin

Ingredients:

- 1 cup sugar
- ½ cup sunflower or olive oil
- 6 drops chamomile essential oil
- 2 drops neroli essential oil
- 4 drops rose essential oil

Directions:

Step 1: Mix the sugar and all the oils together in a small metal bowl.

Step 2: Once completely mixed, transfer the body scrub into an airtight glass jar.

Body Scrub for Acne

While acne is the bane of almost every teenager's existence, it is not limited to your youth. In fact, middle-aged men and women experience an outbreak every once and awhile. This body scrub helps naturally clear up the acne no matter which body part it appears on.

Ingredients:

- 1 cup finely ground oats
- ½ cup water
- 10 drops cypress essential oil
- 10 drops lemon essential oil
- 5 drops lavender essential oil

Directions:

Step 1: Combine the oats and water together in a small mixing bowl.

Step 2: Add the essential oils to the oatmeal and water mixture. Incorporate all the ingredients together.

Step 3: Store the homemade acne body scrub in an airtight container.

Step 4: To use, gently massage the body scrub over the areas where acne is a problem. Rinse the body scrub off your skin and pat dry with a towel.

Ginger and Orange Foot Scrub

This foot scrub is wonderful for those rough areas of your feet. Not only will it help smooth your feet, but it works wonders when rubbed on calluses.

Ingredients:

- ½ cup white sugar
- 2 tablespoons olive oil
- 6 drops orange essential oil
- ½ teaspoon ground ginger

Directions:

Step 1: Pour the white sugar and ground ginger into a mixing bowl.

Step 2: Mix the two dry ingredients together with a metal spoon.

Step 3: Drizzle the olive oil and essential oil over the dry ingredients. Mix once again with a spoon.

Step 4: Transfer the foot scrub from the mixing bowl into an airtight container. Store in the fridge for up to 2 weeks.

Tips: You can substitute 1 tablespoon of orange juice if you don't have orange essential oil. Keep in mind, however, that you won't receive the health benefits that come with the essential oil.

Detox Body Scrub

Epsom salt – one of the ingredients in this scrub – contains magnesium, which helps to draw toxins out of your body and relieve joint pain. Applying this detox body scrub once a week is a great way to cleanse your body from the harmful toxins you are exposed to on a daily basis.

Ingredients:

- 1 cup Epsom salt
- 1 cup Organic coconut oil

Directions:

Step 1: Mix the two ingredients together in an airtight container. Before taking a bath, lay a towel out flat on the bathroom floor. Fill the bathtub up to the desired amount of water. Disrobe and stand on the towel.

Step 2: Rub the detox scrub over your dry body in a gentle motion. Any excess scrub should land on the towel. Remember to rub the scrub all over your body, from your neck to your ankles. Avoiding getting the scrub on your feet as the oil can increase the chance of a slip and fall.

Step 3: Carefully step in the bathtub and slip into the water. Let soak for about 15 minutes before rinsing the scrub off your body. Carefully step out of the bathtub and dry with a towel.

Invigorating and Muscle Pain Relieving Salt Scrub

Ingredients:

- 1 cup sea salt
- ½ cup coconut oil
- 5 drops lavender essential oil
- 5 drops eucalyptus essential oil
- ½ teaspoon ground cinnamon

Directions:

Step 1: Dump the sea salt in a glass mixing bowl. Pour the coconut oil over the salt.

Step 2: Mix the salt and oil together with a wooden spoon. Add the essential oils and cinnamon and stir once again with a wooden spoon.

Step 3: When ready to use, rub the body scrub over sore muscles. Let the scrub sit on the area for several minutes before rinsing it off with warm water.

Sugar, Spice and Everything Nice: Body Scrub Recipes for Women

While these recipes may have a more feminine theme to them, anyone can enjoy the benefits that the homemade body scrubs provide.

Pink Grapefruit Body Scrub

Ingredients:

- 3 cups fine granulated sugar
- ½ cup of pink grapefruit juice (squeezed from a fresh grapefruit)
- ½ cup safflower oil
- 15 drops grapefruit essential oil (optional)
- 10 drops vitamin E oil (optional)

Directions:

Step 1: Mix the sugar, grapefruit juice and safflower oil together in a bowl.

Step 2: Add the grapefruit essential oil and vitamin E oil. Mix all the ingredients together.

Step 3: Store the grapefruit body scrub in the fridge for up to 2 months.

Green Tea and Mint Body Scrub

Ingredients:

- 1 cup sugar
- 3 tablespoons Epsom salts
- 2 tablespoons light olive oil
- 2 tablespoons honey
- 2 green tea bags
- 2 mint tea bags
- 6 drops spearmint essential oil
- 4 drops vitamin E oil (optional)

Directions:

Step 1: Combine the sugar and salt together in a small mixing bowl.

Step 2: Open the 4 tea bags and dump the contents into the bowl. Mix all the dry ingredients together with a spoon.

Step 3: Add the honey and olive oil. Mix with a spoon.

Step 4: Add the essential oil and vitamin E oil. Mix again with the spoon.

Step 5: Store the green tea and mint body scrub in an airtight container. When ready to use, rub the scrub over your dry skin before taking a bath or shower. Rinse the scrub off with water.

Cherry Blossom Body Scrub

Ingredients:

- 1 cup granulated sugar
- ½ cup canola or olive oil
- 2 to 3 drops cherry blossom essential oil
- 5 to 10 drops red soap colorant (optional)

Directions:

Step 1: Mix the sugar and olive oil together in a storage container.

Step 2: Add the cherry blossom essential oil and soap colorant. Mix thoroughly for several seconds until well incorporated.

Step 3: Store the body scrub in a cool, dry place until ready to use.

Mandarin Body Scrub

Ingredients:

- 2 mandarin oranges
- 1 cup coconut oil
- ½ cup sugar

Directions:

Step 1: Remove the peels from the mandarin oranges. Place the peels in a blender or food process and finely chop. Set aside for the moment.

Step 2: Combine the coconut oil and sugar together in a airtight container.

Step 3: Add the chopped mandarin orange peels and stir with a spoon.

Step 4: Attach the lid to the container and store in a dry, cool location.

Pineapple Sugar Body Scrub

Ingredients:

- 1 ½ cup white sugar
- ½ cup coconut oil
- ½ of a pineapple

Directions:

Step 1: Puree ½ of a pineapple in a food processor until it has a smooth consistency.

Step 2: Scoop out ½ cup of the pureed pineapple and dump inside a mixing bowl.

Step 3: Add the sugar and oil and mix thoroughly.

Step 4: Spoon the pineapple body scrub into a sealable container.

Mango and Oats Body Scrub for Sensitive Skin

Ingredients:

- 1 fresh mango
- 2 tablespoons oats
- 1 teaspoon honey

Directions:

Step 1: Cut the mango into pieces and place them in a food processor or blend to puree.

Step 2: Transfer the pureed mango into a sealable container.

Step 3: Add the oats and honey. Mix with a spoon for several seconds until well combined.

Step 4: Place the lid on the container and store in a cool, dry location until ready to use.

Creamy Chocolate Cake Body Scrub

Ingredients:

- 1.5 ounce coconut oil
- 1 ounce shea butter
- .25 ounce sweet almond oil
- .5 ounce cocoa butter
- .25 hemp seed oil
- .35 ounce sunflower oil
- .5 ounce cyclomethicone
- .3 ounce white kaolin clay
- .25 ounce chocolate devils food cake fragrance oil
- 1 ounce vanilla buttercream fragrance oil
- 12 ounce white sugar
- 1 teaspoon xanthum gum powder
- 1 tablespoon diamond dust mica

Directions:

Step 1: Melt the cocoa butter, shea butter and coconut oil together in a double boiler.

Step 2: Remove from heat and add the hemp seed oil, sweet almond oil, sunflower oil, fragrance oils and cyclomethicone.

Step 3: Mix the sugar, xanthum gum powder and mice together in the sealable storage container.

Step 4: Pour the melted oils into the sugar mixture and whisk together with a fork.

Step 5: Store the body scrub in a cool location until ready to use.

Peach and Sugar Body Scrub

Ingredients:

- 1 cup white sugar
- ½ cup olive oil
- 2 to 4 drops peach essential or aromatherapy oil
- 5 to 10 drops of peach soap colorant (optional)

Directions:

Step 1: Mix all the ingredients together in a glass jar. Make sure it is well combined.

Step 2: Secure the lid on the glass jar and place in a dry, cool location when not in use.

Orange Creamsicle Body Scrub

Ingredients:

- 2/3 cup brown sugar
- 1/3 cup olive oil
- 10 drops vitamin E oil
- 5 drops vanilla extract
- 5 drops orange essential oil
- 1 tablespoon honey (optional)

Directions:

Step 1: Mix the brown sugar and olive oil together in a mixing bowl.

Step 2: Add the vitamin E oil, vanilla extract and essential oil, mixing thoroughly.

Step 3: Mix in the honey. You can skip this step but honey is wonderful for dry skin.

Step 4: Store the orange creamsicle body scrub in an airtight container.

Raspberry and Sugar Body Scrub

Ingredients:

- 1 cup white granulated sugar
- ½ cup oil, such as olive, coconut or sweet almond
- 2 to 3 drops of raspberry aromatherapy oil

Directions:

Step 1: Mix all three ingredients together in a plastic or glass sealable storage jar.

Step 2: Store the raspberry and sugar body scrub in a dry, cool location.

Mango Paradise Body Scrub

Ingredients:

- ½ cup raw sugar

- 2 tablespoons coconut oil

- ¼ cup raw mango, chopped

- 3 to 4 drops orange essential oil

Directions:

Step 1: Blend the sugar with the coconut oil in a mixing bowl.

Step 2: Add the chopped raw mango and mush it into the sugar/oil mixture.

Step 3: Add the orange essential oil. Blend all the ingredients together.

Step 4: Store the mango paradise body scrub in an airtight container.

Lavender and Tangerine Body Scrub

Ingredients:

- ½ cup sugar
- ½ cup kosher salt
- 85 drops tangerine essential oil
- 35 drops lavender essential oil
- ¼ cup avocado oil
- ½ cup almond oil

Directions:

Step 1: Combine the sugar and salt together in a mixing bowl.

Step 2: Add the avocado and almond oil and mix thoroughly with a spoon.

Step 3: Add the essential oils and mix again with the spoon.

Step 4: Transfer the body scrub in an airtight container and keep in a dry, cool location.

Moisturizing Body Scrub

Ingredients:

- ½ cup shea butter
- 3 tablespoons olive oil
- 3 teaspoons coconut oil, melted and cooled
- ½ cup brown sugar

Directions:

Step 1: Dump the shea butter into a small pan. Heat the butter on low heat until it is soft but not melted.

Step 2: Transfer the softened shea butter to a mixer and mix on high speed until it develops a whipped consistency. This will usually occur within 4 minutes of mixing.

Step 3: Mix the melted coconut oil and olive oil together in a small bowl.

Step 4: Pour the oil mixture into the mixing bowl containing the shea butter.

Step 4: Use the mixture to mix the oil and butter together for 1 to 2 minutes.

Step 5: Add the brown sugar and mix gently by hand with a wire whisk.

Step 6: Store the body scrub to an airtight container.

Margarita Body Scrub

Ingredients:

- ½ cup salt
- 2 tablespoons olive oil
- 1 to 2 tablespoons tequila
- Juice from 1 lime

Directions:

Step 1: Combine all the ingredients together in a mixing bowl until a paste forms. If needed, add a bit more olive oil.

Step 2: Store the body scrub in an airtight container.

Step 3: Before bathing, rub the scrub over your body. Carefully, step into the bathtub and rinse the scrub off.

Mojito Body Scrub

Ingredients:

- 3 tablespoons granulated sugar
- 1 tablespoon grapeseed oil
- 1 tablespoon jojoba oil
- 4 drops peppermint essential oil
- 8 drops lime essential oil

Directions:

Step 1: Mix the grapeseed oil, jojoba oil and granulated sugar together in a small bowl.

Step 2: Add the essential oils and mix for several seconds.

Step 3: Transfer the body scrub into an airtight container and store in a cool, dark place.

Vanilla and Cinnamon Oatmeal Body Scrub

Ingredients:

- ¾ cup brown sugar
- ¾ cup white sugar
- ¾ cup oats
- ½ cup coconut oil
- ¼ cup olive oil
- 1/2 teaspoon ground cinnamon
- 1 teaspoon pure vanilla extract

Directions:

Step 1: Pulse the oats in a food processor until they have a texture similar to course sugar.

Step 2: Place the coconut oil in a pan and heat on low until the coconut oil melts. Alternatively, melt the coconut oil in a microwave.

Step 3: Combine all the ingredients together in a mixing bowl.

Step 4: Scoop the body scrub into the desired storage container. Keep in a cool, dry place until ready to use.

Citrus Body Scrub

Ingredients:

- 1 cup course sea salt
- ½ cup sugar
- ½ cup coconut oil
- 10 drops sweet orange essential oil
- 10 drops grapefruit essential oil
- 5 drops lemon essential oil

Directions:

Step 1: Combine the salt and sugar together in an airtight jar.

Step 2: Melt the coconut oil on low heat. Once it becomes a liquid, remove the oil from heat.

Step 3: Pour the melted coconut oil over the salt/sugar mixture.

Step 4: Add the essential oil. Don't stir the ingredients!

Step 5: Let cool to room temperature before securing the lid on the container and placing in a cool, dry location until ready to use.

Ginger and Coconut Oil Scrub

Ingredients:

- ¼ cup coconut oil
- 1 tablespoon coarsely chopped ginger
- ¼ cup sweet almond oil
- ¾ cup granulated sugar
- ¼ cup salt, kosher

Directions:

Step 1: Place the coconut oil and ginger in a saucepan. Heat the ingredients on low for 5 to 10 minutes until the oil becomes liquefied.

Step 2: Place a strainer over an airtight container. Pour the liquefied mixture into the strainer to remove the ginger pieces.

Step 3: Add the sweet almond oil to the mixture and stir with a spoon.

Step 4: Stir in the sugar and salt. Attach the lid to the container once the mixture reaches room temperature. Store in a cool, dry location.

Sweet and Spicy Body Scrub

Ingredients:

- 1 cup granulated sugar
- 1 cup brown sugar
- ¾ hazelnut oil
- 2 teaspoons ginger
- 2 teaspoons nutmeg
- 2 teaspoons cinnamon

Directions:

Step 1: Blend the two sugars together in a bowl.

Step 2: Add the ginger, nutmeg and cinnamon to the sugar mixture. Mix with a spoon.

Step 3: Slowly pour the hazelnut oil over the mixture. Use a spoon to combine the oil and dry mixture together.

Step 4: Store in an airtight glass container.

Almond and Orange Body Scrub

Ingredients:

- Handful of almonds
- 1 orange peel
- 1 cup grapeseed oil

Directions:

Step 1: Add the 3 ingredients into a food processor or blend.

Step 2: Blitz the ingredients together until a thick, gritty mixture forms.

Step 3: Scoop the body scrub into a storage container. Keep the container in a dry and cool place.

Chocolate and Coconut Scrub

Ingredients:

- ½ cup brown sugar
- ½ cup granulated sugar
- ½ cup coconut oil
- ¼ cup cocoa

Directions:

Step 1: Combine the brown sugar and granulated sugar together in a storage container.

Step 2: Add the cocoa and mix with a spoon until well blended.

Step 3: Drizzle the coconut oil over the dry ingredients. Mash the mixture together with a spoon or fork until the oil is distributed thoroughly.

Citrus and Green Tea Body Scrub

Ingredients:

- 3 cups Epsom salt
- 3 tablespoons baking soda
- 4 tablespoons apricot kernel oil
- 1 green tea bag
- 8 drops orange essential oil
- 8 drops lime essential oil
- Zest from orange, lemon or lime

Directions:

Step 1: Pour the Epsom salt and baking soda into a mixing bowl.

Step 2: Open the green tea bag and dump the contents into the bowl.

Step 3: Use a fork or spoon to mix the dry ingredients together.

Step 4: Add the oil into the mixing bowl. Mix with a fork or spoon.

Step 5: Add the essential oils and zest. Mix once again with the fork or spoon. The mixture should have a consistency similar to damp packing snow.

Step 6: Transfer the body scrub into the desired storage container.

Chai Masala Body Scrub

Ingredients:

- ¼ cup black tea leaves
- 1 tablespoon ground cinnamon
- 1 tablespoon ground ginger
- ½ teaspoon ground cloves
- ½ teaspoon ground cardamom
- ½ teaspoon ground nutmeg
- ¼ teaspoon ground black pepper
- 1 teaspoon vanilla extract
- 1 cup sugar
- ½ cup coconut oil

Directions:

Step 1: Place the black tea leaves into a coffee grinder and grind into a powder.

Step 2: Dump the ground black tea into a mixing bowl.

Step 3: Add the spices and sugar. Mix with a fork.

Step 4: Mix in the vanilla extract and coconut oil.

Step 5: Store the body scrub in a sealed jar. Use within 3 months.

Java Mint Body Scrub

Ingredients:

- ½ cup coffee grounds
- 2 peppermint tea bags
- ½ cup sugar
- ½ cup coconut oil

Directions:

Step 1: Dump the coffee grounds and sugar into a mixing bowl.

Step 2: Open the peppermint tea bags and empty the contents into the mixing bowl.

Step 3: Add the coconut oil and combine all the ingredients together.

Step 4: Transfer the body scrub to an airtight container.

Almond Joy Body Scrub

Ingredients:

- ½ cup almonds
- ½ cup granulated sugar
- 1 tablespoon cocoa powder
- 1 tablespoon unsweetened coconut flakes
- ½ cup coconut oil

Directions:

Step 1: Ground up the almonds in a food processor. Alternatively, replace the ground almonds with ½ cup of almond meal.

Step 2: Combine all the dry ingredients an airtight storage container.

Step 3: Pour the coconut oil into the container and mix thoroughly.

Step 4: Place the almond joy body scrub in a cool, dry location. Use within three months.

Whipped Grapefruit and Mint Body Scrub

Ingredients:

- ½ cup white sugar
- ½ cup coconut oil
- 1 grapefruit zest
- 1 tablespoon grapefruit juice
- 25 drops grapefruit essential oil
- 10 drops peppermint essential oil
- ¼ teaspoon beet juice (optional)

Directions:

Step 1: Secure the paddle attachment to a stand mixer.

Step 2: Add the coconut oil and sugar into the mixing bowl. Whip the ingredients together on low speed for several minutes until the mixture develops a thick paste-like consistency.

Step 3: Add the zest, juices and essential oil. Mix for a few more seconds until fluffy and well blended.

Step 4: Store the whipped body scrub in an airtight container. It will last longer will stored in the refrigerator.

Lemon and Poppy Seed Cookie Scrub

Ingredients:

- 4 lemons
- 1 cup sugar
- 1 tablespoon poppy seeds
- 1 teaspoon vanilla extract
- ¼ cup cornmeal
- ½ cup coconut oil

Directions:

Step 1: Zest the four lemons. Let the zest dry on paper towels for up to 2 hours.

Step 2: Mix the sugar, poppy seeds, cornmeal, zest and vanilla together in a bowl.

Step 3: Drizzle the coconut oil over the ingredients and mix until well combined.

Step 4: Store the scrub in a sealed jar. Use within 3 months.

Cucumber Sugar Body Scrub

Ingredients:

- 1 cucumber
- 3 cups extra fine granulated sugar
- ½ cup grapeseed oil

Directions:

Step 1: Puree half a cucumber in a food process.

Step 2: Add the pureed cucumber, granulated sugar and grapeseed oil into a mixing bowl.

Step 3: Incorporate the ingredients into one another with a spoon or fork.

Step 4: Transfer the cucumber body scrub to an airtight jar and store in the fridge.

Pomegranate Body Seed

Ingredients:

- 1 cup coconut oil
- ½ cup sugar
- ½ package pomegranate seeds

Directions:

Step 1: Puree the pomegranate seeds in a blender. The mixture will be chunky.

Step 2: Combine the oil, sugar and pureed pomegranate seeds together in a storage container.

Step 3: Attach the lid to the storage container. Keep the pomegranate body scrub in a cool, dry place when not in use.

Sleepytime Bath Scrub

Ingredients:

- 2.5 cups white sugar
- ¼ cup baby oil
- ¼ cup baby bedtime wash
- 4 drops blue food coloring
- 6 drops red food coloring

Directions:

Step 1: Mix the sugar, oil and bedtime wash together ingredients together in a glass jar.

Step 2: Add the food coloring and mix with a fork.

Step 3: Secure the jar closed and place in a cool, dry location.

Step 4: Before your bedtime bath, rub the scrub over your body and rinse off with warm water.

Raspberry and Lemon Sugar Body Scrub

Ingredients:

- ½ cup granulated scrub
- ¼ cup coconut oil, melted
- ¼ teaspoon raspberry extract
- ¼ teaspoon lemon extract
- 1 to 2 drops red food coloring (optional)

Directions:

Step 1: Combine all the ingredients together in a mixing bowl. The body scrub should have a gritty texture.

Step 2: Transfer the sugar scrub into a glass jar where you will keep it until ready to use.

Step 3: Place the jar into the freezer for about 30 minutes. This will allow the scrub to set to the desired consistency.

Step 4: Remove the jar from the freezer and place in a cool location until ready to use.

Apricot Sugar Body Scrub

Ingredients:

- 4 ounces apricot oil
- 1 cup granulated sugar
- A few drops of orange soap colorant (optional)

Directions:

Step 1: Mix the apricot oil and soap colorant together in a bowl. When adding the colorant, do so one drop at a time, stirring after each drop until you achieve the desired color.

Step 2: Add the sugar and stir together with a fork.

Step 3: Store the homemade sugar scrub in an airtight container.

Birthday Sugar Scrub

Ingredients:

- 2.5 cups sugar

- ¼ cup baby wash

- ¼ cup baby oil

- Candy sprinkles

Directions:

Step 1: Mix the sugar, baby wash and baby oil together in a bowl.

Step 2: Transfer the birthday scrub into a glass jar.

Step 3: Sprinkle the candy sprinkles on top of the scrub. These sprinkles are just for decorations.

Step 4: Secure the lid on the jar and keep in a dry, cool place until ready to use.

Herbal Body Scrub

Ingredients:

- 1 cup fine sugar or fine sea salt
- ½ cup sunflower oil
- ¼ cup honey
- 1 vanilla bean, split and scraped
- 10 drops of peppermint essential oil
- 1 teaspoon vanilla extract (optional)

Directions:

Step 1: Mix the sugar or salt with the sunflower oil in a small bowl.

Step 2: Add the honey, vanilla bean, peppermint essential oil and vanilla extract. Stir thoroughly for several seconds until all ingredients are combined.

Step 3: Transfer the body scrub into the glass jar it will be stored in.

Raspberry Lemonade Body Scrub

Ingredients:

- 4 ounces coconut oil, melted
- .5 ounce sesame oil
- 6 ounces white sugar
- .3 ounce raspberry lemonade fragrance oil

Directions:

Step 1: Combine all the ingredients in a glass bowl.

Step 2: Use a fork to whip the ingredients together until well combined.

Step 3: Scoop the raspberry lemonade body scrub out of the glass bowl and into a sealable glass jar.

Step 4: Seal the jar with its lid and store in a cool, dark and dry location.

Snips and Snails and Puppy Dogs Tails: Body Scrub Recipes for Men

Body scrubs are not just for women. In fact, the following body scrub recipes are tailored for the men in your life. These scrub recipes omit the floral and more feminine ingredients often found in commercial body scrubs.

Simple Yet Manly Brown Sugar Scrub

Ingredients:

- 1 cup brown sugar
- ½ cup sweet almond oil (olive oil can be used as a substitute)
- 30 drops of essential oil

Directions:

Step 1: In a small mixing bowl, combine the brown sugar, sweet almond oil and essential oil together.

Step 2: Once well mixed, transfer the manly brown sugar scrub into an airtight container and store in a cool, dry location for about a month.

Tips: When choosing the essential oil, stay away from floral scents – such as lavender or rose – and instead use sandalwood, allspice, cypress, basil, vanilla, black pepper or other more masculine scents.

Face Moisturizer and Exfoliant for Men

Ingredients:

- 2 tablespoons ground oatmeal
- ¼ cup sea salt
- 1 teaspoon water
- ½ teaspoon olive oil
- ½ teaspoon honey

Directions:

Step 1: Combine all the ingredients together in a mixing bowl.

Step 2: Stir the ingredients together until a paste forms. If it is too thick, add a bit more water until you achieve the desired consistency.

Step 3: Transfer the scrub to an airtight container.

Step 4: When ready to use, scoop some of the scrub out of the container with your fingertips and rub it over your face in a gentle, circular motion. Rinse your face with warm water and pat dry with a towel.

Coffee Body Scrub for Men

Ingredients:

- ¼ cup brown sugar
- ¼ cup sea salt
- ¼ cup coffee grounds
- ½ cup olive oil or coconut oil
- 20 to 30 drops of an essential oil, such as vanilla, oakmoss, sandalwood, ginger, basil, balsam or spruce

Directions:

Step 1: Combine the sugar, salt and coffee grounds together in a mixing bowl.

Step 2: Add the oils to the dry ingredients and stir until all ingredients are incorporated into one another.

Step 3: Store the scrub in an airtight container. When ready to use, scoop the scrub out of the container with your hands. Rub the scrub all over your body in a gentle, circular motion. Rinse the scrub off with warm water and dry with a towel.

Pepper and Mint Body Scrub

Ingredients:

- 1 cup Epsom salt
- ½ cup olive oil
- 6 drops mint essential oil
- 1 teaspoon ground pepper

Directions:

Step 1: Mix the Epsom salt and ground pepper together in a small bowl.

Step 2: Pour the olive oil and essential oil over the dry ingredients. Mix all together with a metal spoon.

Step 3: Store the body scrub in an airtight glass jar.

Blood Orange and Vanilla Body Scrub for Men

Ingredients:

- 2 cups white sugar
- ¾ cup coconut oil
- 1 blood orange
- 10 drops vanilla essential oil

Directions:

Step 1: Use a juicer to squeeze the juice from the blood orange into a bowl. Set aside for the moment.

Step 2: Mix the sugar and oil together in a separate mixing bowl.

Step 3: Pour the blood orange juice over the sugar/oil mixture. Use a fork to mix the ingredients together.

Step 4: Add the vanilla essential oil and mix with a fork.

Step 5: Store the blood orange and vanilla body scrub in an airtight container.

Wild Orange and Frankincense Sugar Scrub

Ingredients:

- 1 cup granulated sugar
- ½ cup sweet almond oil
- 8 drops wild orange essential oil
- 6 drops frankincense essential oil

Directions:

Step 1: Pour the sugar in a mixing bowl.

Step 2: Add ½ cup sweet almond oil and stir with a spoon. If necessary, add a bit more oil until you achieve the desired consistency.

Step 3: Add the essential oils and mix again with the spoon.

Step 4: Store the sugar scrub in an airtight container. When ready to use, scoop some of the scrub out of the container with your hand and rub it over your body in a circular motion. Rinse the scrub off with water.

Mint Java Body Scrub for Men

Ingredients:

- ½ cup coffee grounds
- ½ cup white sugar
- ¼ cup hot water
- ¼ cup sweet almond oil
- 20 drops peppermint essential oil

Directions:

Step 1: Mix the coffee grounds and white sugar together in a small mixing bowl.

Step 2: Slowly pour the hot water over the ingredients and mix with a spoon. Let sit undisturbed for 10 minutes.

Step 3: Add the sweet almond oil and essential oil to the mixture.

Step 4: Mix all the ingredients together with the spoon.

Step 5: Transfer the body scrub to an airtight container and store in a cool place.

Coffee Sugar Scrub for Men

Ingredients:

- 1 cup of regular ground coffee
- 1 cup white sugar
- ½ cup olive oil
- 1 tablespoon ground cinnamon
- 1 teaspoon ground nutmeg

Directions:

Step 1: Mix all the ingredients together in a bowl.

Step 2: Transfer the mixture into a glass, airtight container.

Step 3: Lightly rub the scrub over damp skin. Rinse the scrub off the skin and pat dry with a towel.

Mud Scrub for Men

Ingredients:

- 1 cup sugar, brown or white
- 5 tablespoons fresh coffee grounds
- ¼ cup oil, olive or almond
- 1 teaspoon vanilla extract

Directions:

Step 1: Mix the sugar and coffee grounds together in a bowl.

Step 2: Add the oil to the mixture until a paste begins to form.

Step 3: Add the vanilla extract and mix with a spoon.

Step 4: Store the mud scrub in an airtight container until ready to use.

Irish Cream Sugar Body Scrub

Ingredients:

- 1 cup granulated sugar
- 1 tablespoon dry milk
- ½ cup coconut oil
- 2 to 4 drops peppermint essential oil
- 2 to 3 drops green food coloring

Directions:

Step 1: Mix all the ingredients together, starting with the dry ingredients and ending with the liquid ingredients.

Step 2: Transfer the homemade body scrub into an airtight jar and place in a dry, dark and cool area.

Sage and Sea Salt Scrub

Ingredients:

- 2 cups fine sea salt
- 1 cup olive oil
- 4 to 6 fresh sage leaves
- ½ cup date sugar
- 1 red or white grapefruit

Directions:

Step 1: Pour the olive oil and fresh sage leaves into a blender. Puree the two ingredients together for about a minute on high.

Step 2: Mix the salt and sugar together in a bowl.

Step 3: Pour the puree mixture over the salt/sugar mixture and mix together with a spoon.

Step 4: Add a bit of the grapefruit zest into the mixture and stir once again with a spoon.

Step 5: Store the body scrub in an airtight container when not in use.

Irish Coffee Body Scrub

Ingredients:

- ½ cup sugar
- ½ cup fresh coffee grounds
- ½ cup nut oil
- 2 to 3 drops mint essential oil

Directions:

Step 1: Mix the sugar and coffee grounds together in an airtight container.

Step 2: Add the nut oil and mix thoroughly with a spoon.

Step 3: Add the mint essential oil one drop at a time. Mix once again with the spoon.

Step 4: Secure the lid onto the container and place in a dry location away from direct heat and direct light.

For the Little Ones: Body Scrubs Safe for Children

While most ingredients in body scrubs are not harmful to children, some essential oils can pose a risk since the dilution rate is usually low in the body scrub. Eucalyptus, rosemary and peppermint are just a few of the essential oils that are potentially dangerous for children. To prevent accidents, avoid using body scrub on children 10 years old or younger. And if you are ever in doubt, consult with a doctor about which essential oils are completely safe for your little ones.

Pink Body Scrub

Ingredients:

- ½ cup white sugar
- 1 cup honey
- 1 teaspoon strawberry essential oil
- ½ teaspoon pure vanilla extract
- 4 tablespoons baby oil
- 2 drops pink food coloring

Directions:

Step 1: Mix all the ingredients together in a mixing bowl.

Step 2: Transfer the pink body scrub into a sealable container or jar.

Step 3: Store the pink body scrub in a dark, cool and dry location.

Oatmeal and Tea Body Scrub

Ingredients:

- Chamomile tea bag
- 6 tablespoons water
- 1 cup old fashioned oats
- 2 tablespoons honey

Directions:

Step 1: Fill a mug with 6 tablespoons of boiling water.

Step 2: Seep the chamomile tea bag in the water for 5 to 10 minutes.

Step 3: Remove the tea bag from the mug and let cool to room temperature.

Step 4: Pour the oats into a mixing bowl. Add the cooled tea to the oats and let sit for a few minutes.

Step 5: Add the honey and mix thoroughly until well combined.

Step 6: Store the body scrub in an airtight container in the fridge.

Citrus Sweet Scrub

Ingredients:

- ½ cup granulated sugar
- 4 tablespoons honey
- 3 tablespoons orange juice

Directions:

Step 1: Mix the sugar and honey together in a bowl.

Step 2: Add the orange juice. Combine with a fork.

Step 3: Transfer the citrus sweet scrub into a storage container until ready to use.

Changing with the Season: Holiday Themed and Seasonal Body Scrub Recipes

Using the same body scrub recipe over and over again can become mundane rather quickly. So why not switch it up a bit and create homemade body scrubs that match the current holiday or season!

Pumpkin Spice Latte Scrub

Ingredients:

- 1 ½ cups brown sugar
- 2 heaping tablespoons of instant coffee
- 2 tablespoons pumpkin pie spice
- ¾ to 1 cup of sweet almond oil

Directions:

Step 1: Pour the brown sugar in a mixing bowl. Use a spoon or fork to break up any clumps.

Step 2: Add the coffee and pumpkin pie spice to the brown sugar. Mix with a spoon or fork.

Step 3: Pour the oil over the dry ingredients. Use the fork or spoon to incorporate the brown sugar, coffee, spice and oil together.

Step 4: Transfer the pumpkin spice latte body scrub into an airtight container. Use within 2 months.

Tips: Don't fret if you don't have pumpkin pie spice on hand or cannot find it in the stores. You can simply make your own by combining 3 teaspoons ground cinnamon, 2 teaspoons ground ginger, 1 ½ teaspoons ground cloves and 1 ½ teaspoons ground allspice.

Pumpkin Spice Sugar Scrub

Ingredients:

- 2 cups brown sugar
- ½ cup white sugar
- 1 teaspoon ground cinnamon
- 1 teaspoon pumpkin pie spice (see alternative in the recipe above)
- ½ teaspoon nutmeg
- ½ cup sweet almond oil or coconut oil

Directions:

Step 1: Mix the sugar and spices together, making sure to break up any lumps.

Step 2: Pour the oil over the mixture slowly, stirring the ingredients together with a metal spoon. If the scrub is too dry, add a bit more oil. But remember, you don't want the scrub to be runny. It should have a damp texture.

Step 3: Mix all the ingredients together for several seconds. Once thoroughly mixed, transfer the pumpkin spice sugar scrub into an airtight container. Store in the refrigerator for up to 8 weeks.

Autumn Spice Body Scrub

Ingredients:

- ¼ cup brown sugar
- ¼ cup white sugar
- 2 tablespoons powdered ginger
- 2 tablespoons ground cinnamon
- 2 tablespoons powdered nutmeg
- 2 tablespoons powdered cardamom
- 1 cup sweet almond oil

Directions:

Step 1: Pour all the dry ingredients into the airtight glass jar you will store the body scrub in.

Step 2: Drizzle the sweet almond oil over top the dry ingredients. Carefully mix all the ingredients together with a metal spoon.

Step 3: When ready to use, wet skin and rub a small amount – about the size of a half dollar – in a circular motion over your skin. Rinse with lukewarm to warm water. Pat dry with a towel.

Pumpkin Spice Facial Scrub

Ingredients:

- ½ cup white sugar
- ½ cup brown sugar
- ¼ cup pumpkin puree
- ½ teaspoon pumpkin pie spice
- ½ teaspoon vitamin E oil

Directions:

Step 1: Mix the two sugars together in a bowl. Add the pumpkin pie spice and mix again.

Step 2: Mix the pumpkin puree and pumpkin pie spice into the dry ingredients.

Step 3: Transfer the homemade pumpkin body scrub into an airtight container until ready to use.

Hot Chocolate Sugar Body Scrub

Ingredients:

- 3 tablespoons cocoa powder
- 1 cup light brown sugar
- 1 teaspoon vanilla extract
- ½ cup olive or sweet almond oil

Directions:

Step 1: In a small mixing bowl, combine the cocoa powder, light brown sugar and vanilla extract.

Step 2: Add the oil and mix until thoroughly combined.

Step 3: Store the hot chocolate sugar body scrub in a sealable jar.

Holiday Spice and Brown Sugar Scrub

Ingredients:

- 1 cup of brown sugar
- ½ cup sweet almond oil
- 4 bags of spice herbal tea

Directions:

Step 1: Pour the brown sugar in a mixing bowl.

Step 2: Open the 4 bags of spice herbal tea and dump the contents into the mixing bowl.

Step 3: Use a metal spoon to mix dry ingredients together.

Step 4: Drizzle the oil over the dry ingredients and mix together with the spoon.

Step 5: Store the spice and brown sugar scrub in an airtight glass jar for 1 to 2 months.

Tips: If you cannot find spice herbal tea, use 1 teaspoon cinnamon, 1 teaspoon ginger, 1 teaspoon nutmeg, 1 teaspoon cocoa powder, ½ teaspoon clove, ½ teaspoon cardamom, dash of black pepper and ½ teaspoon vanilla extract. If you don't have a spice on hand, just leave it out of the recipe. The scrub will still smell lovely and work just as good.

Winter Facial Scrub

Ingredients:

- ¼ cup oats, finely ground
- 1/3 cup white rice flour
- 1/8 cup shredded coconut, finely ground
- 1 tablespoon neem powder
- 1 tablespoon kaolin clay
- 2 tablespoons calendula, finely ground
- 2 tablespoons chamomile, finely ground
- 15 drops rose hip seed oil
- 10 drops rose essential oil
- 10 drops chamomile essential oil

Directions:

Step 1: Use a food processor to finely grind oats, shredded coconut, calendula and chamomile. Dump the ingredients into a mixing bowl.

Step 2: Add the remaining dry ingredients (white rice flour, neem powder and kaolin clay) to the mixing bowl. Mix with a wooden spoon.

Step 3: Add the oils to the dry ingredients, stirring after each type of oil is added.

Step 4: When ready to use, dump about 1 teaspoon of the scrub in the palm of your hand. Add a few drops of water and mix with your finger. Apply the paste to your face and lightly scrub for a few minutes. Rinse your face with water and pat dry with a towel.

Step 5: Store the winter facial scrub in an airtight container for 6 to 12 months in a cool, dry location.

Rosemary and Mint Infused Holiday Sugar Scrub

Ingredients:

- 1 ½ cup turbinado sugar (also known as raw sugar)
- 1/2 cup avocado oil
- 1 tablespoon dried or fresh rosemary
- 1 tablespoon dried or fresh peppermint
- 1 tablespoon nettle leaves
- ½ cup shea butter

Directions:

Step 1: Pour the avocado oil in a small saucepan.

Step 2: Add the herbs – rosemary, peppermint and nettle leaves – to the oil-filled saucepan.

Step 3: Place the pan on your stove. Turn the heat on the lowest setting and let heat for about 30 minutes.

Step 4: Remove the pan from the heat and let cool to room temperature.

Step 5: Place a sieve over an airtight glass jar. Strain the oil through the sieve so the oil is separated from the herbs. Discard the herbs.

Step 6: Wipe the saucepan clean with a towel. Pour the oil back into the clean saucepan. Add the shea butter.

Step 7: Let the butter melt for about 5 to 10 minutes. Remove the saucepan from heat. Let the mixture cool for a few minutes.

Step 8: Pour the sugar into the airtight glass jar. Add the oil/butter mixture and stir all the ingredients together.

Step 9: Store the infused body scrub in a cool, dry location for 1 to 2 months.

Gingerbread Body Scrub

Ingredients:

- 2 cups brown sugar
- 1 cup olive oil (sweet almond oil or coconut oil can also be used)
- 2 tablespoons ground ginger
- 2 tablespoons pumpkin pie spice
- 1 tablespoon honey or vitamin E oil (optional, but recommended for dry skin)

Directions:

Step 1: Dump the brown sugar in a mixing bowl. Break up any clumps in the sugar with a spoon or fork.

Step 2: Add the spices to the brown sugar and stir for several seconds until well incorporated.

Step 3: Pour the olive oil and honey or vitamin E oil over the dry ingredients. Stir with the spoon or fork for several minutes.

Step 4: Scoop the gingerbread body scrub out of the mixing bowl and into an airtight container. Store in a cool, dry place until ready to use.

Candy Cane and Brown Sugar Scrub

Ingredients:

- 4 cups brown sugar
- 1 cup almond oil
- 1 cup olive oil
- 5 drops peppermint essential oil
- ½ teaspoon vanilla extract

Directions:

Step 1: Mix all the ingredients until well blended.

Step 2: Transfer the body scrub into an airtight container.

Step 3: When ready to use, rub the scrub over your body massaging it into the skin. Rinse off with lukewarm water and dry with a towel.

Chocolate and Peppermint Body Scrub

Ingredients:

- 3 cups white sugar
- ½ cup cocoa powder
- 1 cup coconut oil
- 1 ½ teaspoon peppermint essential oil

Directions:

Step 1: Melt the coconut oil in a double boiler. Remove from heat.

Step 2: In a separate bowl, mix the sugar and cocoa powder until thoroughly combined.

Step 3: Pour the melted coconut oil over the sugar/cocoa mixture and combine with a spoon.

Step 4: Add the peppermint essential oil and mix with the spoon.

Step 5: Spoon the body scrub into a sealable glass jar. Store in a cool, dry room until ready to use.

Summer Scrub

Ingredients:

- 1 cup sea salt
- 1 cup raw sugar
- 1 cup coconut oil
- 30 drops sweet orange essential oil

Directions:

Step 1: In a glass jar, add the sea salt and sugar. Use a butter knife to carefully combine the two ingredients together.

Step 2: Add the coconut oil and stir once again with the butter knife.

Step 3: Add the sweet orange essential oil. Use the butter knife to carefully mix all the ingredients together.

Step 4: Store in a cool, dry place until ready to use.

End-Of-Summer Tomato Sugar Scrub

Ingredients:

- 2 cups granulated sugar
- 1 large tomato, chopped
- ¾ cup olive or coconut oil
- 5 to 20 drops lemon or citronella essential oil

Directions:

Step 1: Chop the tomato into fine pieces until it almost has a mush consistency.

Step 2: Pour the sugar in a mixing bowl. Add the chopped tomato. Stir the two ingredients together.

Step 3: Pour the oil slowly over the sugar/tomato mixture.

Step 4: Blend the ingredients together with a spoon.

Step 5: Add the essential oil and blend the ingredients together once again.

Step 6: Transfer the tomato sugar scrub to an airtight container. Store in the fridge until ready to use.

Kissable and Lickable: Homemade Scrub Recipes for Lips

Wind, moisture, sun and even the foods and drinks you consume can take a toll on your lips leaving them cracked, dry and less than desirable. Regular use of the following lip scrub recipes can greatly increase your kisser.

Cinnamon and Sugar Lip Scrub

Ingredients:

- ½ tablespoon raw sugar
- 1 ½ tablespoons brown sugar
- 2 tablespoons cinnamon oil
- Drop of vanilla extract

Directions:

Step 1: Combine the 4 ingredients together in a mixing bowl. Work the ingredients into one another using a fork or spoon.

Step 2: Transfer the lip scrub into the desired container.

Step 3: When ready to use, scoop a small amount of the cinnamon and sugar lip scrub out of the container with your fingers. Rub the scrub gently over your lips in a circular motion. Wipe off with a damp cloth.

Tip: Leave the cinnamon and sugar lip scrub on overnight for smoother lips.

Natural and Nourishing Lip Scrub

Ingredients:

- 1 tablespoon honey
- 1 tablespoon brown sugar
- 1 tablespoon olive oil

Directions:

Step 1: Combine all the ingredients together in a mixing bowl. Transfer the lip scrub to an airtight container.

Step 2: When ready to use, gently rub a small amount of the scrub over your lips.

Step 3: Let the scrub sit on your lips for a minute or two before wiping it off your lips with a damp cloth. Or you could simply lick it off.

Lime and Coconut Lip Scrub

Ingredients:

- 1 tablespoon coconut oil
- 1 tablespoon lime juice
- 1 teaspoon honey
- 3 tablespoons granulated sugar

Directions:

Step 1: Mix the coconut oil, lime juice and honey together in a small bowl.

Step 2: Add the white sugar to the mixture 1 tablespoon at a time. Mix thoroughly after adding each tablespoon of sugar.

Step 3: Store the lime and coconut lip scrub in an airtight container.

Step 4: When ready to use, run the lip scrub over your lips in a gentle, circular motion for several seconds to a minute. Wipe the scrub off your lips with a damp cloth. Repeat once a day for softer, healthier lips.

Honey and Lemon Lip Scrub

Ingredients:

- 1 teaspoon honey
- Dash of lemon
- 1 teaspoon coconut oil
- 2 tablespoons granulated sugar

Directions:

Step 1: Mix all the ingredients together in a glass dish.

Step 2: Dip a soft-bristled toothbrush into the scrub, using the brush to scoop a small amount of the scrub out of the glass dish.

Step 3: Use the toothbrush to rub your lips gently with the scrub. Wipe your lips clean with a damp cloth.

Step 4: Store unused portions of the scrub in an airtight container.

Pumpkin Pie Lip Scrub

Ingredients:

- 2 tablespoons coconut oil
- 1 tablespoon honey
- 1 tablespoon brown sugar
- 1 teaspoon pumpkin pie spice

Directions:

Step 1: In a small bowl, mix the 4 ingredients together.

Step 2: Scoop the pumpkin pie lip scrub into a container and store in a dry, cool spot.

Step 3: When ready to use, rub the scrub across your lips in a gentle back and forth motion. Wipe the excess off your lips with a damp towel.

Simple Coffee Lip Scrub

Ingredients:

- 1 part coffee grounds
- 1 part olive oil

Directions:

Step 1: Mix the two ingredients together until they form a soft paste.

Step 2: Rub a small amount of the coffee lip scrub across your lips in a circular motion.

Step 3: Wipe the scrub off with a cloth.

Step 4: Store any remaining coffee lip scrub in an airtight container.

Put your Best Face Forward: Homemade Facial Scrub Recipes

While the following scrub recipes are gentle enough for your face, you still should take care when using them. Avoid scrubbing too hard as this could irritate your skin and keep the homemade scrub away from your eyes.

The No-Nonsense Face Scrub for Daily Use

Ingredients:

- ½ cup oats, finely ground
- ½ cup almond meal, finely ground
- Liquid (for oily skin, use witch hazel or water, for dry skin use milk and for any skin type, use rosewater)

Directions:

Step 1: Add the oats and almond meal together in an airtight container. This is the base mixture that you will store in a cool, dry place.

Step 2: When ready to use, measure out 2 teaspoons of the base mixture into a small dish.

Step 3: Add a bit of the liquid of your choice to the base mixture. Mix together with your finger and let the oats soak in the liquid for a few seconds.

Step 4: Scrub your face lightly with the homemade mixture. Rinse the scrub off with warm water and pat your face dry with a towel.

Vanilla and Lavender Face Scrub

Ingredients:

- 1 cup white or brown sugar
- ½ cup almond oil
- ½ teaspoon vitamin E oil
- 15 drops lavender essential oil
- ½ teaspoon real vanilla extract

Directions:

Step 1: Mix the sugar and almond oil together in an airtight container.

Step 2: Add the vitamin E oil, essential oil and vanilla extract to the sugar mixture. Stir thoroughly with a spoon.

Step 3: Store the face scrub in a dry and cool location when not using.

Lemon, Honey and Lavender Face Scrub

Ingredients:

- ½ lemon
- 1 tablespoon honey
- ¼ cup sea salt
- 15 drops essential oil
- 2 teaspoons lavender, dried (optional)

Directions:

Step 1: Mix all the ingredients in a small bowl until well blended.

Step 2: Transfer the face scrub into an airtight container.

Step 3: When ready to use, scoop a bit of the scrub out of the container with your fingers. Massage the homemade scrub gently over your entire face. Rinse the face scrub off your skin with warm water. Dry your face with a towel.

Lavender and Lemongrass Facial Scrub

Ingredients:

- 1 cup fine sea salt or raw cane sugar
- 3 tablespoons virgin coconut oil
- 6 drops lemongrass essential oil
- 1 to 2 tablespoons lavender flowers, crushed

Directions:

Step 1: Pour the salt or sugar into a small mixing bowl.

Step 2: Add the coconut oil and mix with a spoon. Add the lemongrass essential oil and mix once again.

Step 3: Sprinkle the crushed lavender flowers over the mixture. Use a spoon to incorporate the crushed flowers into the scrub.

Step 4: Store the facial scrub in a dry, cool place when not using.

Sweet Orange Facial Exfoliant Scrub

Ingredients:

- Orange peel (available in the herb section of health food stores)
- Fine yellow cornmeal

Directions:

Step 1: Combine equal parts yellow cornmeal and orange peel in a container.

Step 2: When ready to use, mix a bit of the exfoliant scrub with your favourite facial cleaner. Gently rub your face with the scrub in a gentle circular motion.

Step 3: Rinse the scrub off and pat your face dry.

Step 4: Store the orange peel and cornmeal mixture in an airtight container.

Oatmeal Facial Scrub

Ingredients:

- 1 cup ground oatmeal
- 1 teaspoon ground rosemary (available in the herb section of grocery stores)
- Ground cinnamon
- Purified water

Directions:

Step 1: Mix the three dry ingredients together in an airtight container.

Step 2: In the morning, scoop out 1 to 2 teaspoons of the dry ingredients and dump it in a small dish.

Step 3: Add water ¼ teaspoon at a time until you achieve a paste.

Step 4: Rub the oatmeal facial scrub gently in a circular motion over your face. Dampen a cloth with warm water and wipe the scrub off your face.

Step 5: The dry ingredients will keep in the airtight container for 6 months if stored in a cool, dry location.

Honey and Oatmeal Facial Scrub

Ingredients:

- ½ cup oatmeal
- 2 tablespoons honey
- 1 teaspoon nutmeg
- 15 drops tea tree essential oil
- 15 drops lavender essential oil
- 1 teaspoon dried lavender (optional)

Directions:

Step 1: Grind the oatmeal up a bit in a blender without making it too powdery. Dump the ground oatmeal into a mixing bowl.

Step 2: Add the nutmeg, honey, dried lavender and essential oils into the oatmeal-filled mixing bowl. Blend all the ingredients together with a spoon.

Step 3: Transfer the facial scrub into a sealable container. Place the container in the bathroom where you can use it on a daily basis. It will keep for 2 weeks.

Don't Forget the Feet: Recipes for Homemade Foot Scrub

These scrub recipes are perfect for dry, cracked and unruly feet. Apply the scrub directly to the tops and bottoms of your feet and rub in a back and forth motion. Don't overlook those rough spots! When finished, rinse the foot scrub off your feet and pat dry with a towel.

Dirty Feet Scrub

Ingredients:

- 1 cup granular sugar
- Dish soap
- 5 drops lemon essential oil

Directions:

Step 1: Pour the sugar into an airtight container that you will be storing the dirty feet scrub in.

Step 2: Add the dish soap one drop at a time until you achieve the desired consistency.

Step 3: Add the lemon essential oil and mix with a spoon. Store in a cool, dry place until ready to use.

Soothing Lavender Foot Scrub

Ingredients:

- 1 cup Epsom salt or sea salt
- ½ cup olive or sweet almond oil
- 8 drops lavender essential oil
- 2 tablespoons lavender buds, dried

Directions:

Step 1: Pour the salt and dried lavender buds into a mixing bowl.

Step 2: Add the olive or almond oil and mix thoroughly with a spoon.

Step 3: Add the lavender essential oil to the mixture and stir with the spoon. Dump the dried lavender buds and fold them into the mixture.

Step 4: Scoop the scrub into a jar and store in a cool location.

Strawberry Foot Scrub

Ingredients:

- 2 teaspoons coarse sea salt
- 2 tablespoons extra virgin olive oil
- 8 fresh strawberries

Directions:

Step 1: Pour the salt into a clean mixing bowl.

Step 2: Add the oil to the salt and mix until well combined.

Step 3: Cut the green tops from the strawberries. Cut the strawberries into slices.

Step 4: Add the sliced strawberries to the salt/oil mixture. Mush the strawberries into the mixture until you have a chunky scrub.

Step 5: Store the strawberry foot scrub in an airtight glass jar.

Peppermint Foot Scrub

Ingredients:

- 1 cup granulated sugar
- Coconut oil or olive oil
- Peppermint essential oil

Directions:

Step 1: Pour the sugar into a bowl.

Step 2: Add just enough coconut or olive oil to the sugar so the mixture is damp but not soggy.

Step 3: Add about 3 to 4 drops of peppermint essential oil. Mix with the spoon.

Step 4: Scoop the peppermint foot scrub into the storage container until ready to use.

Lemon Foot Scrub

Ingredients:

- ½ cup oats
- ½ cup cornmeal
- 2 tablespoons salt, sea or table
- 6 drops lemon essential oil
- Water

Directions:

Step 1: Place the oats into a food processor, blender or coffee grinder. Blend the oats until they are a powder.

Step 2: Dump the ground oats into a bowl.

Step 3: Add the corneal and salt to the ground oats and mix with a spoon.

Step 4: Add the lemon essential oil and mix with the spoon.

Step 5: Add water to the mixture one teaspoon at a time until you achieve a gritty paste.

Step 6: Store the lemon foot scrub in an airtight container.

Soothing Magnesium Foot Scrub

Ingredients:

- 1 cup Epsom salt
- ¼ cup olive oil
- 1 teaspoon Castile soap
- 5 to 7 drops lavender essential oil
- 5 to 7 drops vanilla essential oil

Directions:

Step 1: Mix the salt, olive oil and Castile soap together in a small mixing bowl.

Step 2: Add the essential oils one drop at a time. Mix with a spoon.

Step 3: Store in a glass, airtight jar. Use about 1 teaspoon of the scrub per foot.

Simple Foot Scrub

Ingredients:

- ½ cup sugar
- ½ cup Epsom salt
- ½ cup olive oil
- 10 to 15 drops essential oil (optional)

Directions:

Step 1: Mix the sugar, salt and olive oil together.

Step 2: Add the desired essential oil. Lavender, lemon, sandalwood, citrus and peppermint work well for this foot scrub.

Step 3: Store the simple foot scrub in an airtight container.

Mint and Eucalyptus Foot Scrub

Ingredients:

- 2 cups medium or fine ground sea salt
- 1 cup coconut oil
- 15 drops peppermint oil
- 25 drops eucalyptus oil

Directions:

Step 1: Mix the salt and coconut oil together in a glass jar.

Step 2: Add the peppermint oil and eucalyptus oil, and mix all the ingredients together with a spoon.

Step 3: Secure the lid on the jar and keep in a dry, cool place until ready to use.

Thyme and Peppermint Foot Scrub

Ingredients:

- 1 cup granulated sugar
- ¼ cup sweet almond oil
- ¼ teaspoon dried thyme
- 4 to 5 drops peppermint essential oil

Directions:

Step 1: Combine the sugar and almond oil in a mixing bowl.

Step 2: Add the essential oil to the sugar/oil mixture. Stir with a spoon.

Step 3: Sprinkle the dried thyme over the mixture. Use the spoon to distribute the thyme throughout the body scrub.

Step 4: Transfer the scrub to an airtight container.

Stinky Feet Foot Scrub

Ingredients:

- 1/3 cup raw sugar
- 2/3 cup Epsom salt
- 1 ½ tablespoons coconut oil
- ½ tablespoons peppermint, dried
- 4 drops tea tree oil
- 5 to 6 drops peppermint oil

Directions:

Step 1: Combine the sugar, salt and coconut oil together in a small bowl. All the sugar and salt granules must be coated in oil.

Step 2: Add the essential oils and peppermint flakes. Use a fork to mash the ingredients together.

Step 3: Store the foot scrub in a glass, airtight jar.

How to Use Body Scrubs

Body scrubs are simple to use and require little to no preparation. With that in mind, here are some few tips to help ensure you are using body scrubs effectively and safely.

Using Body Scrubs

Body scrubs can be used on both dry and wet skin. However, most users find the scrub is most effective when used on dry skin. Whether using on wet or dry skin, make sure to rub the scrub over your skin in a circular motion. Some body scrubs recommend leaving the mixture on your skin for a few minutes. This gives the ingredients enough time to penetrate into the skin. Even if the scrub doesn't say 'leave on for so many minutes' there is no harm in allowing the scrub to sit on your skin for a few minutes. When you are ready to remove the body scrub, simply rinse it off with lukewarm water.

Unless designed for use on your face, refrain from applying the body scrub to your face and neck. The skin on your face and neck is generally more sensitive than the skin found on other parts of your body, which can lead to irritation.

Body scrubs can be a bit messy and you can cut down on the cleanup process by laying newspaper or a towel down on the floor and then standing on it while applying the scrub. Another option is to stand in the shower while applying the body scrub.

Usually only two or so tablespoons of the body scrub is needed per use. Using too much not only results in waste but also increases the chance for accidents due to slippery surfaces.

Safety Concerns

Since body scrubs are used to exfoliate the skin, you should err on the side of caution and rub the scrub gently. Rubbing too hard could result in irritated, red and painful skin. With that in mind, you shouldn't be alarmed if you start to old layers of dead skin fall off. This is actually one of the benefits of body scrubs.

Since most body scrubs contain oil as a main ingredient, they can make surfaces slippery. This increases the risk of slip and fall injuries.

Your skin absorbs the ingredients in the body scrub. This could become problematic for those who have health conditions that require closely monitoring sugar and salt intake. For those individuals, skip the salt and sugar body scrubs and instead use scrubs with alternative exfoliators.

Gift Giving and Selling

Shelf Life: Prolonging the Shelf Life of your Homemade Body Scrubs

While the shelf life of the body scrub varies depending on the ingredients used, you can help prolong its shelf life by following a few simple rules:

- Keep the homemade scrub in an airtight container. It doesn't matter if it's glass or plastic, just make sure to always store the homemade body scrub in an airtight container.
- Store the homemade scrub in a cool and dry location. Keeping the unused body scrub in a cool and dry location is essential to prolonging its life.

Some recipes recommend storing the body scrub in the fridge. This is usually not necessary if you store the body scrub properly. If you decide to keep your body scrub in the fridge, it may begin to set up. This can be corrected by simply sitting the body scrub on your kitchen container for about 20 to 40 minutes before use. Once the scrub reaches room temperature, stir it with a fork or spoon.

Storage: Choosing the Right Container for Body Scrubs

While any airtight container can successfully store your homemade body scrub, you should think outside the box if giving away or selling them. Avoid plain, square containers and instead use small individual jars made from glass or plastic. Jars with locking bail lids are perfect for body scrubs. They come in various sizes, are airtight and the locking lid is conveniently attached to the jar.

Mason jars and jelly jars are another option for your body scrub and can often be found at grocery and department stores. Mason jars are sometimes less expensive than bail lid jars, which make them the more economical choice.

For lip scrubs, however, consider something a bit smaller. Glass or plastic cosmetic containers designed for lip balms work great for your homemade lip scrub and give it a more professional look.

The Devil is in the Detail: Preparing the Body Scrubs for Presentation

While you can simply fill the desired jar with the body scrub and hand it to the person, why not take the extra steps to dress it up a bit. No matter how amazing it is, if the outward appearance doesn't match, your homemade body scrub may not entice the receiver to use it. A simple ribbon tied around the jar can make a big difference in its appearance. But do you really want to stop there? Consider taking things a bit further and putting thought into all the details no matter how small they may seem.

Labels

Labels are relatively inexpensive, come in a wide array of shapes and sizes and can be written or printed on. Furthermore, labels can be customized to fit the season, occasion or your desires. They can also be placed directly on the jar or on the top of the lid.

Scrapbook Paper

Scrapbook paper works great for covering up those unattractive lids and is available in a wide array of prints and designs. Simply place the lid on top of the paper and trace around it, adding about ¼-inch around the edge. Use a pair of sharp scissors to cut the shape out and then glue it onto the lid. The edges of the shape will need to be pushed down inside the lid and secured with glue.

Scraps of Fabric

Like the scrapbook paper, fabric can be used to cover ugly jar lids. The edge of the fabric can be attached to the inside of the lid – like you would do with the scrapbook paper – or simply tied to the exterior of the lid to create a more rustic or cottage feel.

Stickers

While you're browsing the scrapbooking aisle, take a look at the stickers used to decorate scrapbooks. These stickers can be attached to the jar to spruce it up a bit. Just don't overdo it and instead stick to simple yet elegant stickers, such as decorative swirls. Adding too many stickers will cause the jar to look cluttered and messy.

Paint

Hand painting is another option to dress up ho-hum jars. However, this is usually more time consuming than other decorating options.

Include the Recipe

Another option is to print or neatly write the ingredients and directions for the body scrub on a label that you attach to the jar. This will provide the person receiving the scrub all the information they need to make their own batch.

Conclusion

No matter what your reasoning for making body scrubs, just have fun and experiment with the recipes. If you don't have a certain ingredient on hand and don't want to take a trip to the store, simply substitute it! Just make sure you have an exfoliant and carrier oil and your body scrub should still work great.

Printed in Great Britain
by Amazon.co.uk, Ltd.,
Marston Gate.